RONNIE O'SULLIVAN

with Rhiannon Lambert

TOP OF YOUR GAME

70 Recipes To Help You Eat For Success

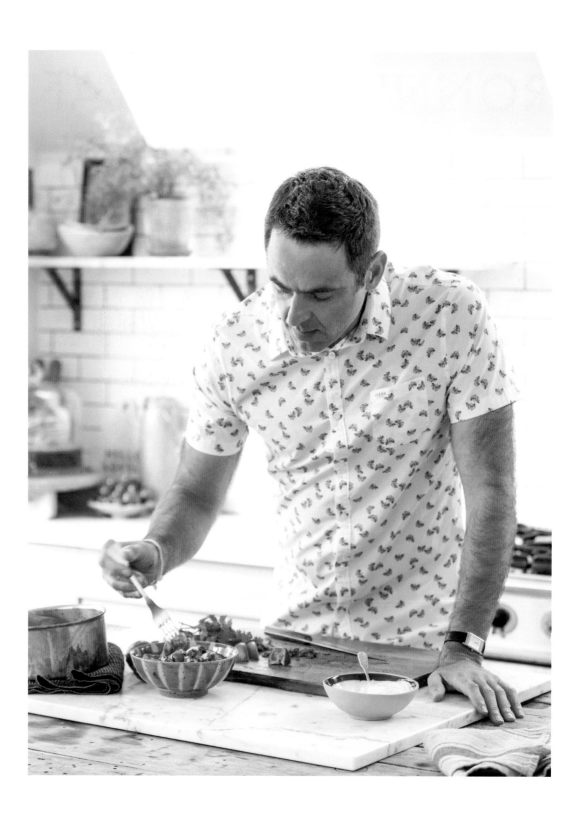

RONNIE O'SULLIVAN

with **Rhiannon Lambert**

TOP OF YOUR GAME

70 Recipes To Help You Eat For Success

Published by Lagom
An imprint of Bonnier Books UK
The Plaza,
535 Kings Road,
Chelsea Harbour,
London, SW10 0SZ

www.bonnierbooks.co.uk

Paperback 9781788700917
eBook 9781788701181

A CIP catalogue of this book is available from the British Library.

Printed and bound by Graficas Estella in Spain

1 3 5 7 9 10 8 6 4 2

Lagom is an imprint of Bonnier Books UK
www.bonnierbooks.co.uk

CONTENTS

INTRODUCTION 09

MINDSET 27

WHAT IS ON YOUR PLATE? 71

RECIPES 105

BREAKFAST 107

LUNCH 147

DINNER 173

ON-THE-GO SNACKS 203

INDEX 216

AUTHOR BIOS 220

ACKNOWLEDGEMENTS 224

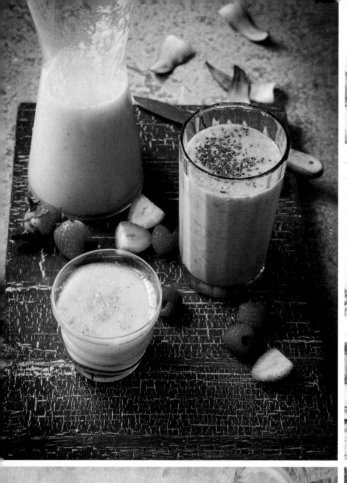

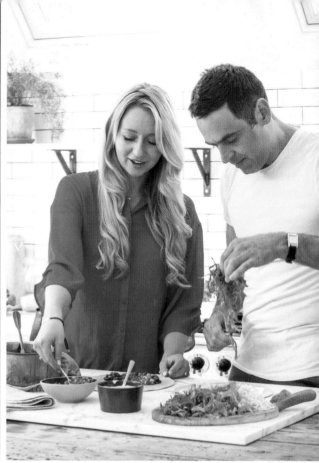

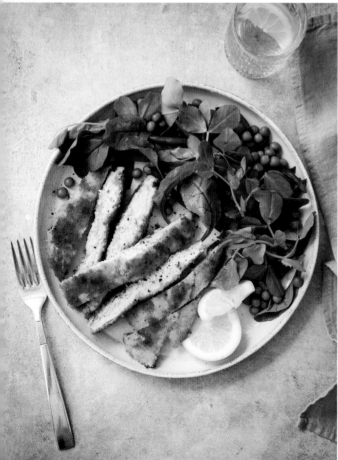

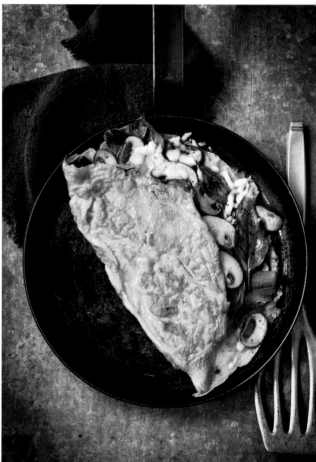

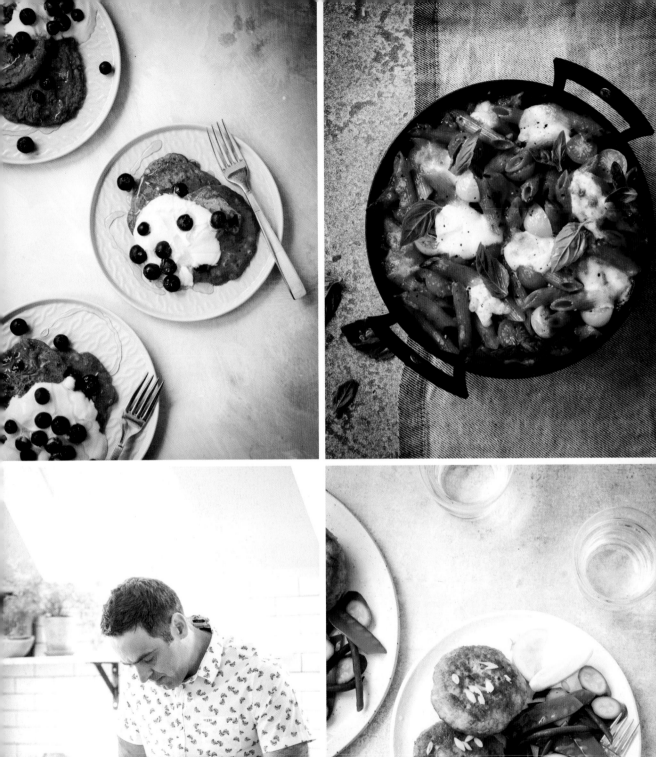
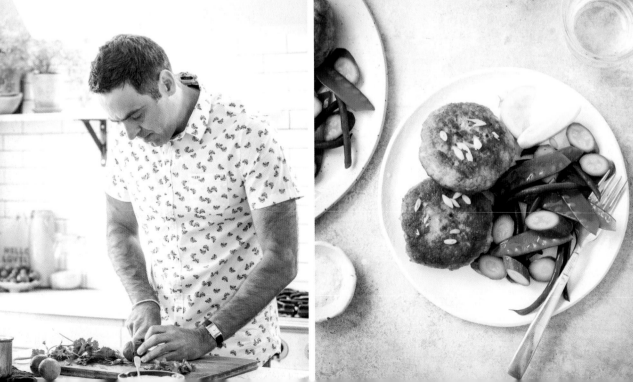

INTRODUCTION

INTRODUCTION

You might well be thinking, 'Why is the world snooker champion Ronnie O'Sullivan telling me how eating well will change my life? He isn't a chef – he wins snooker championships, so what does he know about food?'

These are all questions that I wouldn't blame you for asking as you think about buying this book – after all, moderation, healthy living and self-care aren't necessarily things that you would automatically associate with me. I've been very honest about my addictive personality in the past; depending on the year and what else was going on in my life, my addictions have included drink, drugs, food, Prozac and running. It's taken me a while, but I can now accept that my addictive personality is just the way I am – it's my nature and I'm finally okay with that.

But I've also learned to manage that nature by changing my diet and regarding food as the fuel that can help me get the best out of life. The idea that what you put in dictates what you get out is not rocket science, but I now realise that what's on my plate has a massive impact on how I feel and, most importantly, on how I play snooker. I don't want you to pick this book up and think, 'Oh here we go, another person in the public eye is telling me to buy expensive "healthy" food, when he probably has people to cook for him.' I actually look after myself and try to keep my life simple and focused with good food and good exercise, which (I hope) helps me play my best. All this also makes me nice to be around and helps me to be a better dad too. That's all I care about.

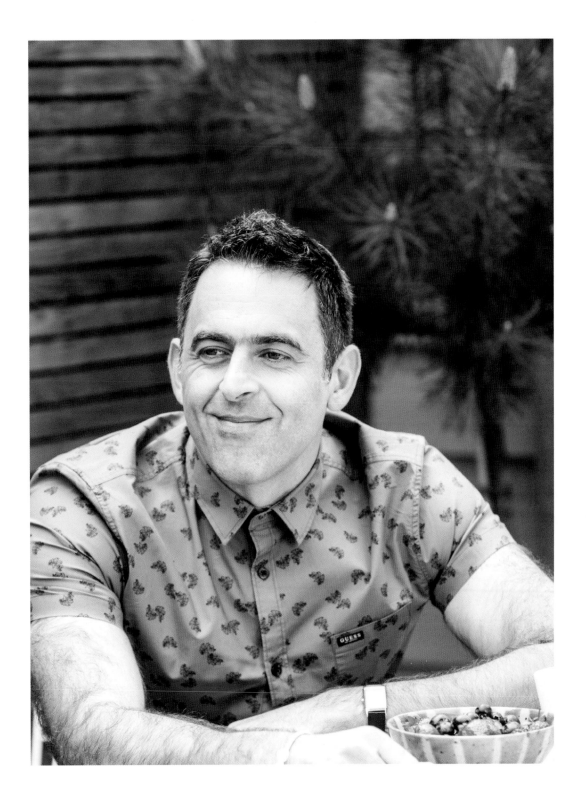

Being motivated to be the best is what drives all ambitious people. I'm never satisfied with myself and want to be as good as I can. That said, though we all love to win, I genuinely believe that as long as you do your best and try to improve, it's doesn't matter where you finish. There's nothing wrong with coming last, as long as you've given yourself the best chance and are curious about how you can do even better next time.

Whatever sport or business you're in, you should always be looking around at your competitors and asking, 'Is anyone doing anything better than me? And can I learn from them?' Since I sorted out the way I eat, I have more belief that I might be able to play for a bit longer than I previously thought. I'd love to think I could still be competing and winning tournaments well into my fifties – and who knows? What I do know is that it all comes down to how I treat my body and my mind.

As you will learn in this book, my new addiction is a really healthy one: it's a commitment to eating well that is making me feel the best I ever have. I've finally realised that my body needs to be nourished rather than punished and that, if I look after it in the right way, it will do right by me. It sounds obvious but it's true – you get out what you put in and the machine is only as good as the fuel you use. To be the very best at what you do, you need to invest in yourself – it's all about being motivated to reach your full potential in whatever you do. Be proud of the talent and skills you have, but also know that you have to do your bit. I know from experience that nothing comes to you just because you want it.

I hope this book will help you realise that life is all about moderation. Thinking about food this way has shown me that I can still have the odd fry-up if I make better choices; I'll have rye bread, two eggs, two pieces of halloumi, avocado and tomatoes, but won't have the unhealthy bacon or sausages. It's still delicious and it's still a treat – and it shows what I'm trying to do in this book. It isn't about denial – it's about finding the option that suits you best and making healthy changes.

It takes a lot of hard work and dedication to maintain the level of excellence needed to consistently win world snooker tournaments. At times it used to feel impossible, but since I've been following a healthy eating plan for the last couple of years, all that has changed – my renewed physical energy, mental staying power and self-belief have taken me to the best place of my career. In this book, I really want to show you how you can eat, think and work your way to being number one – and stay there.

This book won't give you an easy way out; if you know you're eating badly, I won't tell you that you can still pile your plate with the terrible food that got you in the state where you need to make changes. You're reading this book because you need to shake things up – we all get into that situation now and again, but the trick is to recognise it and find someone who can set you on the right path. I did some research, and tried to find someone on my wavelength who spoke common sense and could help me understand what I needed to eat in order to get the best out of myself. I found Rhiannon Lambert, a registered nutritionist who specialises in weight management and sports nutrition.

I didn't want to follow just another diet book, which would force me to count calories, avoid a long list of foods and leave me feeling miserable all the time. The months before I started working with Rhiannon had been one long cycle of denial, bingeing, guilt, yo-yo weight loss and instant gratification. I knew that if I wanted to treat my body the way I should and eat in the very best way, I needed to surround myself with the best experts.

Rhiannon and I were introduced on email to start off with, and the first time we met, we talked for hours! I was instantly impressed by her knowledge and just knew that she would help sort me out – I've always believed that we should go straight to the people who know more than us when we need help. They are experts for a reason! Rhiannon runs a clinic in London where she teaches her simple approach to eating well, free from dieting and any kind of restriction. It sounded like it would suit me perfectly.

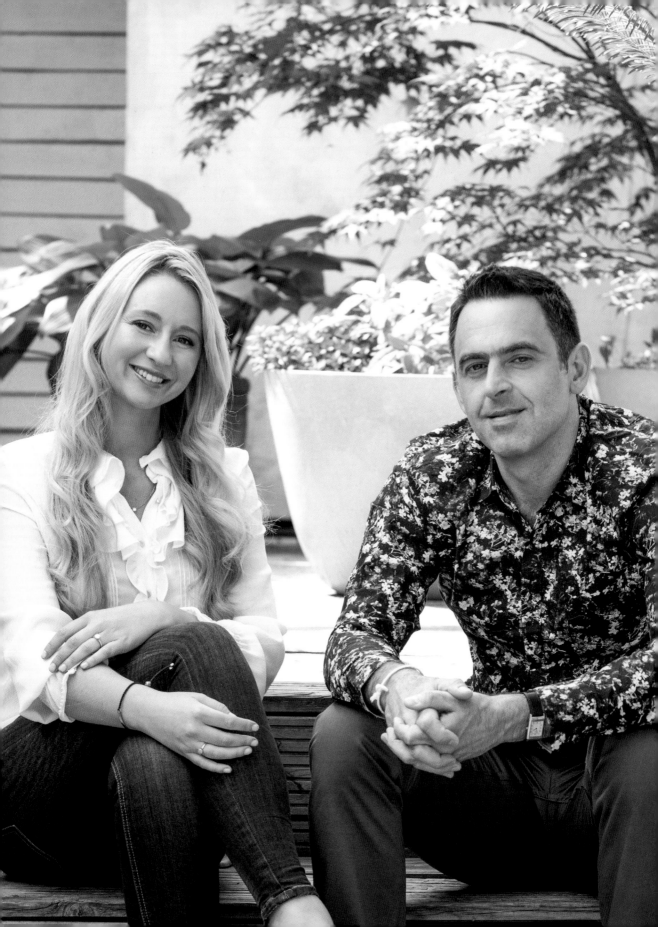

After our first meeting, we scheduled regular appointments; at the first one, Rhiannon sat me down and we talked about my current diet. Once we had done that, she asked me lots of questions and we examined my childhood attitude to food, my food associations and the triggers that set off bad eating habits in me. It wasn't just about what I ate and when – it was also about why I ate, what I did, and the feelings and emotions that were linked to my behaviour. It took a while to get my head around it, but I haven't looked back since then.

Before I met Rhiannon, I'd eat heavy meals that would make me really tired or give me a big spike in energy, followed by a crash. I realise now that it's all about keeping myself topped up and stable, eating regularly without overdoing it. My big problem has always been that I think I need to eat more than I do, so learning when my plate is full enough has been a real game-changer.

This book won't help you make excuses; you can't out-train a bad diet, but neither can you be the best if your body and mind don't have what they need in order for you to be number one. My advice? Set some goals for yourself, and then smash them. You have one life, so why waste it being average when you can learn to be great?

WHAT THIS BOOK WILL GIVE YOU:

An easy-to-follow guide for living better, eating more healthily and helping your brain to enhance your performance, whatever it is you do.

A collection of seriously tasty recipes.

A proper examination of how food links to brain health and can enhance concentration. What you eat can have a massive impact on your mental sharpness, and can also help with problems like insomnia and anxiety. The difference it has made to my snooker has been amazing.

Tips and information about how to eat and train; whether you are on the road all the time like me or sitting at a desk all day, there's always a healthy choice – you just have to train yourself to take it.

Help to cope with the stress of modern life.

"YOU CAN'T
OUT-TRAIN
A BAD DIET"

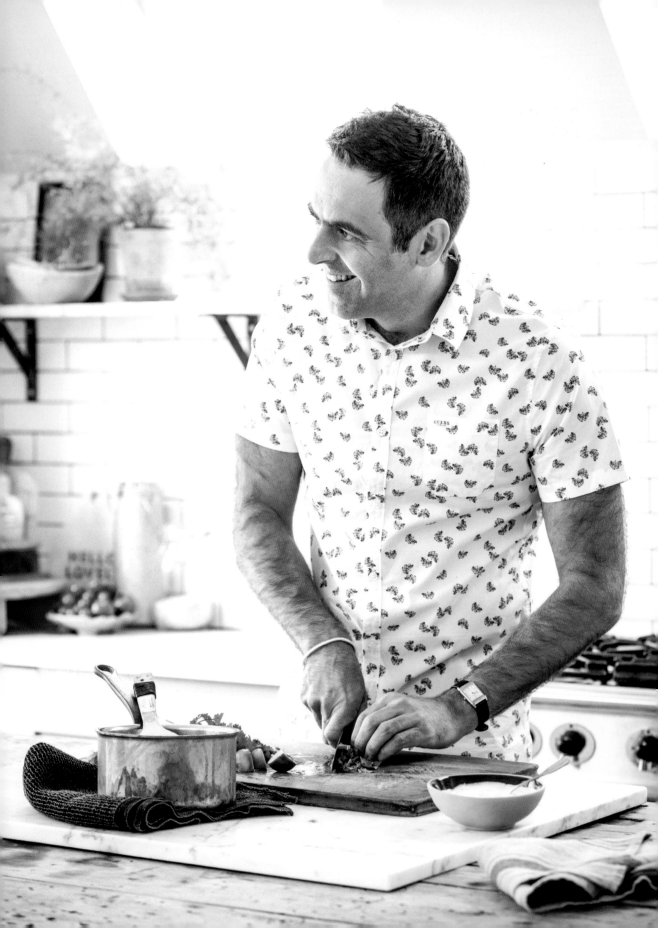

MY FITNESS AND NUTRITION JOURNEY

LEARNING FROM EXPERIENCE

I grew up in an Italian household where food was taken so seriously that it was almost like a religion – the evening meal when we sat down as a family to eat bowls of steaming pasta, delicious casseroles and sweet desserts was the highlight of the day. We would linger over meals and eat much more than we needed to, continuing to pick at the food my mum had lovingly prepared long after we were full. I can't really remember when I became aware that food was one area where I was definitely 'all or nothing', but I think I was a teenager when I realised I had put on some weight.

The public know a lot about my life – how I struggled when my dad went to prison, for instance. I suppose it was around that time that my addictive personality really started to come out, and when I first discovered drink and drugs. I began to feel out of control, and over the years, I've gone down that same road more times than I'd care to admit.

Like most people, I've always known the basics when it comes to nutrition. We all know that a diet of pizza and beer, with loads of takeaways each week, will cause us to pile on the pounds. But if you struggle with doing things in moderation, like I do, that self-knowledge can go completely out the window.

I suppose over the years I've experienced a cycle of getting bigger and feeling crap about myself, and then training excessively, almost as if I was punishing myself. It obviously caused my weight to go up and down like a yo-yo, but more importantly it had the same effect on my mood. This had a direct effect on how I performed in my day job as a snooker player. I always expected a stupid amount from my body, even though I was abusing it – how was I supposed to concentrate for hours on end, when I wasn't giving my body and brain what it needed?

I've always been into fitness and loved running as a teenager, but stopped when Dad got banged up – in fact, I stopped doing everything that was good for me. Looking back, it was the beginning of my all-or-nothing attitude to life.

Once he got out of prison, he was on at me right away to get back into the training – 'no excuses' was his motto, and he was completely right. I had turned professional at 16 and when I started to go running, there was no doubt that my snooker improved. The days were long – I was often picked up at 8am and dropped home after midnight. The key to my success at snooker was staying focused and having the right level of concentration – and running helped me with that.

Although I might not always appreciate it, I'm someone who needs structure and I'm a nightmare when it is disrupted. So when Dad was convicted for murder, my structure was turned upside down and drink and drugs took over my life. Before I knew it, I was 20 years old, weighed over 15 stone, was addicted to pretty much every drink and drug around and was the not-so-proud owner of a 37-inch gut. I was fat, miserable and far from the top of my game. I felt gross and knew that I needed to turn things around.

I started running again and lost three stone. For the next few years, it was the thing that kept me in check. Even when the rest of my life looked like a car crash, it kept me sane, kept my weight steady and allowed me to tell myself I had things under control. The running was a crutch during the shit times and I started doing it competitively in 2004. On the outside, everything looked rosy, especially as I was World Champion, but I was feeling low and trying desperately to stay clean. It was a rocky road that that was full of bumps, stints in The Priory, Narcotics Anonymous meetings and more ups and downs than I can remember.

What I lacked was consistency in any part of my life, and I lurched from one crisis to another, determined to do everything my own way. Lots of snooker players like to do the same thing over and over again, following the same routine and moving slowly and deliberately; I'm the opposite and have always had trouble sitting still, concentrating on what's in front of me and doing what's expected of me. One minute I was 17 years old and winning my first major title; the next I'd been suspended for head-butting an official – that was how my life went.

After a while, I wasn't able to cope with the pressure. When it comes to snooker, even the most basic shot requires a combination of thinking ahead, speed, being precise and a reliance on the laws of science. You spend most of the time trying to control the uncontrollable, which pretty much sums up my whole life! I have talked openly about my love-hate relationship with both the game and myself, and the two things often seem to go together. When I first went off the rails, the snooker table became a complicated place for me to be, with many bad associations.

I won my first tournament at nine years old and it took a long time and hard work to get to the point where I overtook Stephen Hendry's record of 775 century breaks. But in my thirties, the wheels came off everything – I was too in my head and found myself unable to deliver the cue. My manager at the time persuaded me to see Steve Peters, a professor of psychiatry at Sheffield University. He used to be a doctor at Rampton Secure Hospital, but started working with elite athletes to help improve their mental performance. He gave me the ability to do what I needed to get my focus back.

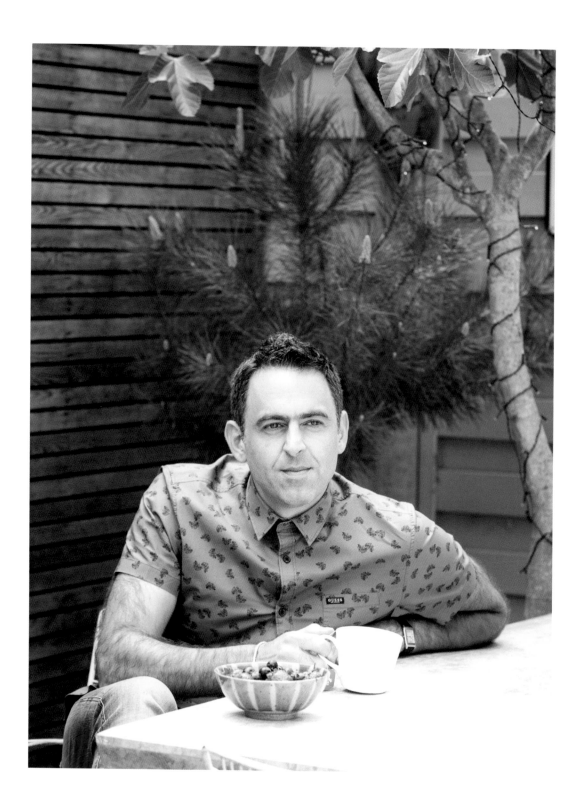

My attitude to running also helped my attitude to snooker. If you run for miles every day of the week, you end up being knackered and not matching your personal best, and it was the same with snooker – before a tournament I would cram in as much training as possible, but would wonder why I was going backwards and getting worse. I realised then that there is such a thing as overdoing it and this means that you don't bring your 'A' game. I know now that we are all beginners at one stage, so the most important thing is trusting yourself and realising that it's all part of the journey to be the best we can be. Don't worry about anyone else and stay focused on your own lane. Let others try to look over your shoulder. They are behind you for a reason.

NO EXCUSES – BE AT THE TOP OF YOUR GAME

We're all good at different things, and there's enough information out there to help you be whatever you want to be. I don't do excuses or half measures and neither should you: if you have bought this book to help you make a change, then don't talk about reading it – just get on and read it! If you want to give up smoking, find the best expert for that, and if you want to give up drugs, do the same thing. When I first decided I wanted to play snooker, I immediately identified Stephen Hendry as the best person I could learn from and used to watch him for hours on end – he was world number one, so I watched him to find out why, and that helped me become the best too.

With anything new I think, 'Who is at the top of their game?' and I say the same thing to the younger players I'm surrounded by now. I often hear them come out with excuse after excuse and blaming bad luck when they lose in a tournament, and I just won't have it. For me, there isn't any such thing as luck or coincidence – it's hard work, focus and determination that help you get to the top and stay there, and it's all about creating the life you want and being the best version of yourself. I now include eating the right food for my body in that list of must-do things. Thinking about food and eating the right things is key to keeping myself on the straight and narrow in every aspect of my life.

You don't have to completely wipe out your old life – it's all about taking steps in the right direction. If you want to train, make the commitment. You don't have to be Mo Farah – just get your heart rate up and stretch your muscles three or four times a week and, as long as you've also sorted your diet, you'll start to see the changes. That's the bit that I didn't have sorted until the penny finally dropped and I realised that you really can't exercise a bad diet away.

MAKING THE CHANGE

Often, he hardest thing is knowing that you need to make a change, but in September 2017, I knew that was what I had to do. I'd hit a wall with my physical and mental wellbeing, and I was fat again, despite the fact that I was over-exercising. Deep down, I knew I was eating way too much of all the wrong things, which meant that despite the exercise, my body was not able to lose any weight.

I needed to rediscover the feeling of being at peak mental and physical health, which meant changing my life in order to get the best out of myself. Everything was suffering: I was playing badly because I was so knackered all the time and I couldn't practise as much as I needed to because I had no energy. I was following a carbohydrate-free diet to try and drop some pounds, without realising that my brain needed good carbohydrates to function during matches. I was literally running on empty, while also expecting an elite performance from my exhausted, starving body.

I know it's all about eating great food, pacing yourself, recuperating and understanding that your mental health is just as important as your physical health. And the biggest gains are made when you fuel yourself well and rest properly – this sort of thinking has changed my life. I treated myself badly back then, because that was how I felt. Now I treat myself like a Ferrari: you can't get me out every day, but when you do, you can be confident that you will get the best, because I'm well looked after in between performances.

I'm an open book in many ways, and particularly when it comes to my relationship with snooker. It's well known that I have a complicated relationship with the game that has made me famous. I've won five World Championships, which places me just behind Steve Davis and Ray Reardon (who have both won six) and Hendry (who has won seven), but despite this success, there have been days when I could hardly look at a cue, when I've had zero motivation and have wanted to quit the game completely. Looking back, so much of that attitude had to do with the fact I wasn't fuelling my mind properly. That's a thing of the past now, and I don't even recognise the old me – the person who couldn't walk anywhere without dripping in sweat and was miserable, and desperate for change. My decision that enough was enough marked a real turning point. As with anything I do, I have to learn it for myself and wade through the facts so that I understand what I am doing and, most importantly, why I am doing it.

In the same way that I wanted to excel at snooker, it was important to me that I excelled at my new regime and got the knowledge I needed to take charge of my life and form new, healthier habits. Rhiannon gave me the knowledge I needed to get going.

MINDSET

MINDSET

Our bodies are amazing things. Sometimes I think about what I've done to mine over the years: how far I've pushed it, how much I expected from it and how little I gave it – after all this, I'm amazed that I'm still standing, never mind still playing! But it wasn't until I started thinking properly about how I treated myself in terms of food that I thought about how amazing the brain is, and how much I rely on it to play my best snooker.

I've had my depression battles over the years, many of which have been pretty public, but the truth is that strong mental health is linked to everything we do, and yet it's often the thing we look after least – that was certainly the case with me. Since I've changed up my diet, I've really started to live by the idea that we can only take care of our long-term physical and mental health when we take a proper look at our diet and lifestyle.

Obviously everyone is different, but I genuinely think that feeding your mind and body properly can help avoid the sorts of dark places that I've found myself in over the years. The trick is to try and avoid getting into a negative cycle, and what we eat can play a massive part in keeping us steady.

MENTAL HEALTH ON A PLATE

The mind is a complicated and finely tuned machine and it needs careful maintenance – we need to keep balanced if we expect it to work to its maximum capacity. You should be able to perform at the highest level, whatever your goals are, and we can make that happen by looking after how we fuel the brain.

We all feel like we're going nowhere at some point in our lives, and I've been no different. When I met Rhiannon in September 2017, it was the start of the new snooker season and my mental ability to play the game was suffering, largely because of my diet. I'd hit a wall and was feeling fed up with everything and not as switched on as usual. Everything felt like a slog – I was in a rut and needed help with my head, my game, and everything else! I needed to play well, with no excuses about a lack of energy or feeling in bad shape.

I immediately liked Rhiannon's positivity – looking back, I definitely needed some of that, given my negative frame of mind. I was properly depressed and was also unable to run due to an injury – over the years, I'd torn ligaments, broken my foot and had numerous calf and Achilles problems. I was literally falling apart, and also used to sweat like a beast, because I was carrying too much weight – Rhiannon must have wondered what she'd let herself in for when I walked into her clinic for my appointment!

HOW DO YOU EAT?

Rhiannon and I immediately set about trying to identify patterns that were particular to how I ate. I wouldn't say I'm greedy, but I love my food and once the training had gone out of the window, so had my self-restraint. Suddenly that cheeky portion of fish and chips and a second pudding felt acceptable and I very quickly let myself go — it was as if without the running, there were no consequences or brakes. I couldn't just have one cheesecake, so I'd have four, while thinking, 'Why can't I stop?'

I'd always thought that some tough training would solve all my issues but, after Rhiannon had analysed what and how I ate, I started to understand that every aspect of my performance was either enhanced or diluted by what I consumed. The key shift was also looking at food in terms of my internal physical and mental health, and not just in terms of how I looked. Writing the evidence down on paper was not a pretty sight and one thing was clear: I needed to get a handle on the situation right away.

RHIANNON: THE MAGIC INGREDIENT IS KNOWLEDGE

Snooker is a sport that involves a great deal of concentration over a long period of time — eating well is extremely important for this and it can really enhance how you think and feel. Without carbohydrates, Ronnie felt tired and not at his best, but as soon as we re-introduced them, his energy levels soared and his brain began to work properly again. Carbohydrates are the brain's preferred source of fuel, so it's no wonder that he felt better after they had been re-introduced into his diet. The fog lifted for Ronnie and he was able to view his game more clearly.

The average person in the UK should aim for 30g of fibre every day. Ronnie and I discussed how we could improve his digestion and also support his gut health, which is linked to maintaining a healthy weight and a happy mind.

BEFORE		AFTER
2 eggs and an avocado	BREAKFAST	Porridge with berries and flaxseed
Chocolate bar or biscuits	SNACK	Fruit and yoghurt
Mezze, including a tub of hummus, falafel, rice, bread and chicken	LUNCH	Chicken, rice and salad
Crisps	SNACK	Hummus, rye crispbreads and cottage cheese
Two portions of curry	DINNER	Fish, sweet potato and vegetables
Chocolate cake	DESSERT	Fruit

MY GOALS:

- Optimum health

- Good digestion

- Support sports performance

- Body fat reduction

EATING FOR MIND

This was the first thing I tackled, as it was the most urgent issue. I couldn't even be bothered to pick up a cue, didn't care if I won or lost and was spending a lot of my time sleeping instead of practising. My first discovery was that when you don't eat enough nutrient-rich foods, your body lacks essential vitamins and minerals, which can have a negative effect on your energy, mood and brain function.

Rhiannon taught me that having the ability to focus and concentrate comes from the supply of glucose that's used by the brain as energy – in fact, the brain uses 20 per cent of all the energy that is supplied to the body! Glucose is also essential to fuel your muscles and maintain a constant body temperature. The glucose in our blood comes from carbohydrates, such as fruit, vegetables, cereals, rice, bread, potatoes, sugars and the lactose in milk.

To play my best snooker game, I had to start making sure my meals were properly balanced and gave me extra glucose, so that my body could store some for an emergency. This would help keep me sharp and keep my temperature calm and my heart steady. Long training sessions and matches that go on for hours cannot be fuelled by sugary energy drinks and bacon sandwiches covered in HP Sauce. My old diet and carb-cutting meant that I didn't have the stamina; a lack of glucose meant I got headaches and felt sweaty, all at a time when I should have been concentrating on finishing off an opponent.

Being on the road makes it harder to keep yourself in line. Long days of playing would often end with a visit to a nice restaurant, and it had always been easy to reward myself with lots of comfort food. What's so brilliant about my healthier lifestyle now is that I can still do that, but instead of ordering a dessert and then finishing off my mate's, I now share one with someone else. I don't feel like I'm depriving myself because I still get a taste – I just don't need all the extra helpings! Best of all, because I'm

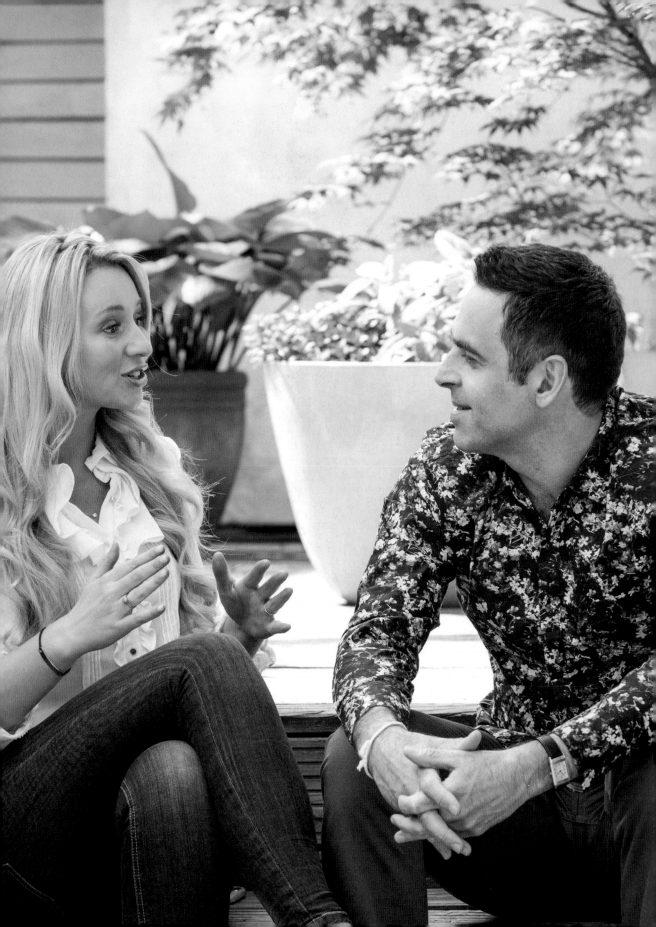

cooking the recipes that Rhiannon gave me, I can look at a menu and know exactly what to choose and how the food has been cooked. I can easily ask for some fish, potatoes and salad, pretty much anywhere I go.

Preparing your own food gives you the ultimate control – in fact, sometimes I make some food for myself before I go out to a restaurant. This means I don't arrive starving and make bad choices – I know that's a trigger for me. Still, I don't beat myself up if I do fall off the wagon, because a bad day doesn't have to turn into a bad week or month – that's not how it works!

It's actually not so much that I deny myself – it's more that I genuinely don't want to feel terrible and now know which foods will do that to me. When I played in The Masters recently, I watched some of the players eat huge egg and bacon sandwiches covered in HP Sauce. I could tell they'd loved every second, and I have to say that right then and there, I'd have done anything to join them! But two minutes later, they felt terrible and had to get up to play their best snooker while feeling bloated and heavy. I was delighted that I hadn't caved! I've come to realise that my performance is slicker when I feel light and bright, and good food does that for me.

The bottom line is that it has a massive impact on the way we feel, and also that our mood can influence the food choices we make. It's all to do with the habits that we make and what we tell ourselves we need.

I can 100 per cent identify with the slippery slope of diets and weight loss. How many times have we all got on the scales to see that we've put on a few pounds, then gone out to a restaurant and thought, 'Sod it,' before ordering two of everything? For me, that was the story of my life before I understood the consequences of such actions.

"PREPARING
YOUR OWN FOOD
GIVES YOU THE
ULTIMATE CONTROL"

When I behaved like that, it wasn't just that the weight went on – it was also that I would look in the mirror and not like what I saw. Mentally, I got into the habit of hating my reflection and always being angry with myself that I couldn't control my eating. It was really hard on my head and also meant that, being on form and playing a good match became tricky. I would eat badly and feel heavy, and then I'd just be fuming that I'd put so much bad stuff into my body. Then I'd be convinced I would have a bad match – and most times, I would.

I now realise that feeling good physically and mentally is the result of having a diet that gives us the right amount of everything, including healthy carbohydrates. If we eat them regularly throughout the day, they ensure that our concentration and mental energy levels stay stable. For me, this means that there are no dips when I'm in the middle of a match. Eating breakfast is also a must, as it can stop cravings later in the day.

In terms of what we actually need, the old-school clichés are true. Just as we were told when we were kids, fruit and vegetables are really important – and oily fish is good for the brain and our mood. If we build our diet around the basics, we can make sure we don't miss anything.

The table opposite is a helpful way to match which vitamins and minerals we might be missing, based on the impact that not getting enough of them has on our mood:

I had to start from scratch – everything I'd been doing previously had to be scrapped and it felt a bit like rebooting a computer. I sat down with Rhiannon and we put together a nutrition plan that would cover all the bases.

The main thing was that I wouldn't feel hungry, because that's something I find really hard. Being hungry is OK, but when I have important matches to play, I don't want to feel this way. This was also where the reality began to hit home. So many people moan that the main thing stopping them from going on a diet is the fact there's so much they can't eat, and I'm not going

MISSING VITAMIN/ MINERAL	EFFECT ON MOOD	FOODS WHICH CAN HELP
IRON	Feeling weak, tired and lethargic all the time.	The risk of anaemia is reduced with adequate iron intake, particularly from red meat, poultry and fish, beans and pulses and fortified cereals. Not drinking tea with meals may also help.
THIAMIN B1, NIACIN B3 OR COBALAMIN B12 (ALL B VITAMINS)	Tiredness and feeling depressed or irritable.	Fortified foods including wholegrain cereals, animal protein foods such as meat/ fish, eggs and dairy.
FOLATE	An increased chance of feeling depressed, particularly in older people.	Folate is found in liver, green vegetables, oranges and other citrus fruits, beans and fortified foods such as yeast extract (marmite) and fortified breakfast cereals.
SELENIUM	An increased chance of feeling depressed and other negative mood states.	Brazil nuts, meat, fish, seeds and wholemeal bread.

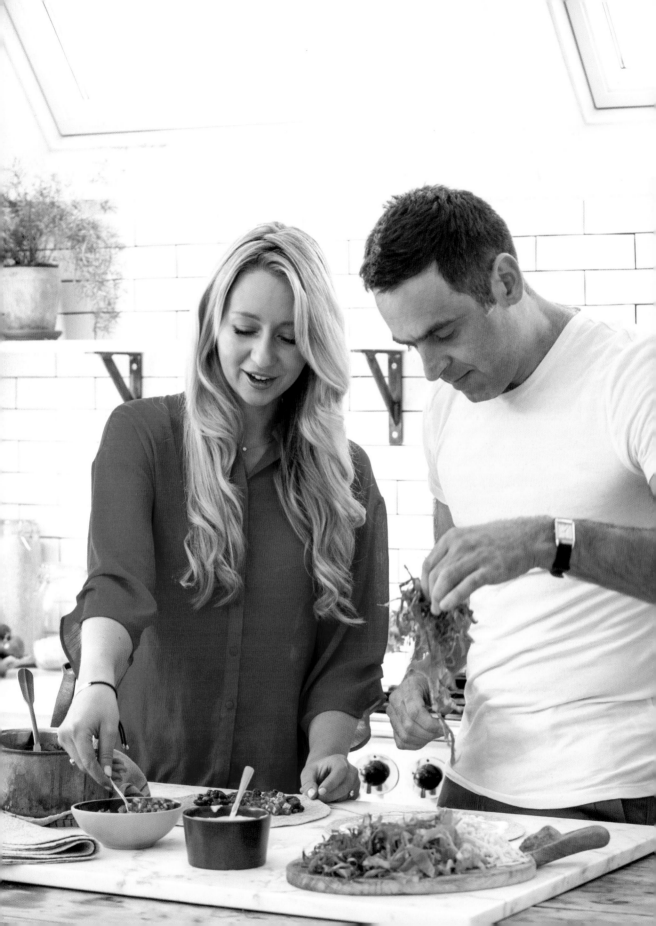

to lie about this – kick-starting a healthy way of living means that a lot of food just has to go, and that's just a fact. I'm not going to pretend that you can have your wine, beer and big bowls of white pasta and still lose weight; you need to want to make the change and stick to it. But I can tell you for a fact, that you won't look back.

BASIC NUTRITION PLAN

> ## BALANCED MEALS = PROTEIN + GRAINS + VEGETABLES + FATS

Most of your meals should be balanced, in order to get the most out of your food and to nourish your body, inside and out.
This requires consistency and you might need to reset your brain –
I certainly needed to challenge my 'all or nothing' mindset.

RHIANNON ENCOURAGED ME TO THINK ABOUT THE FOLLOWING:

- It is possible to eat well on non-running days.

- Why my body needs rest days.

- It is OK to enjoy sugar in moderation.

- You don't have to finish everything on your plate.

- I should try to practise mindful eating: to focus on the smells, textures and flavours of the food while I'm eating, without distraction from technology.

PROTEINS	
For example: chicken, fish, beef, Quorn, cheese, tofu, lentils, beans, chickpeas, eggs, and protein powder	
Chicken	1 breast
White fish	150g when cooked (2 small fillets or 1 large one)
Red meat	70g when cooked (aim to have just once a week)
Oily fish	150g when cooked (approx. 1 fillet)
Beans/pulses	80g or 3 heaped tbsp when cooked
Eggs	2-3
Cheese	30g hard cheese (matchbox sized amount)

GRAINS AND CARBOHYDRATES

For example: quinoa, wholegrain rice, wholegrain pitta, buckwheat, pearl barley, rye bread, amaranth, potato and sweet potato

Grains	75g when cooked (approx. 5-6 tbsp)
Potato	1 medium potato (200g)

FATS

Coconut oil	1 tsp
Extra virgin olive oil	1 tbsp
Olives	8
Avocado	½
Seeds and nuts	1 portion is around 25–30g

VEGETABLES AND FRUIT

Fruit	80g Eat 2-3 portions per day
Vegetables	80g Eat 5 portions per day

TOP TIPS FOR STAYING FOCUSED.

- Almond milk – unsweetened and fortified or semi-skimmed/full-fat dairy milk.

- Reduce tea to twice a day, and then drink herbal teas.

- Aim for two portions of oily fish a week (salmon, mackerel, tuna steak, sardines). Do not exceed four portions in a week.

- Choose leaner meats, fish and vegetarian alternatives over ultra-processed and red meat. Keep red meat to around one meal a week.

- Aim for 2 litres of water a day.

- 2–3 pieces of fruit a day.

- Half an avocado is a portion.

- Limit alcohol intake.

- Try to have some vegetarian meals every week.

AN IDEAL FOOD DAY

An ideal day will look different to everyone, but this really worked for Ronnie. Use the choices on pages 40-41 to build your own ideal food day, or see page 105 for the recipes.

BREAKFAST [8.30AM]

HYDRATE: Wake up, drink a glass of water and then have breakfast when you're ready.

- Porridge or muesli: 60g of oats with unsweetened almond milk or dairy milk, 40g berries and a sprinkling of flaxseed.

- Smoothie: 200ml almond milk, a handful of spinach, 20g oats, 15 frozen grapes (keep a punnet in the freezer for smoothies), 1/2 a banana, 1 inch of fresh ginger, 100g yoghurt, 1/3 cucumber and 1 scoop of protein powder.

- 2 eggs, cooked any way you like, with 1 slice of rye bread and 1/2 an avocado.

SNACK [11AM]

For example:

- 1 small pot of Greek yoghurt (approx. 120g).

- Almonds and a piece of fruit.

- 125g edamame beans.

- 1 apple and 30g nut butter.

- 2 sausages (chicken or vegetarian).

- 2 eggs (if none in the morning).

- Oatcakes or rice cakes, with hummus .

- 1/3 of a tub of hummus (or 2 tbsp) and simple veggie sticks (for example carrot, pepper and cucumber).

- 80g roasted chickpeas with paprika.

LUNCH [1–2PM]

Every lunch should aim to include protein, carbohydrates, vegetables and good fats.

For example;

- 1 fillet of fish, cooked quinoa with vegetable salad and 1 tbsp extra virgin olive oil.

- Tuna with green beans, peppers, garlic, cooked tomatoes, sweet potato and a handful of pine nuts.

SNACK: 4–5PM

Make sure this is different from your morning snack.

DINNER [7–8PM LATEST]

Every dinner should aim to include: protein, vegetables, one portion of carbohydrate and good fats.

If you had chicken at lunch, have fish for dinner, and vice versa – and try to increase your variety of vegetables (like cabbage, pak choi, green beans and spinach) at dinner.

Soups don't have enough protein or carbohydrate in them, so add some on the side!

DESSERT

Remember that you can eat everything in moderation. Pick a dessert you truly love to have once a week and if you fancy something light and sweet on other days, try a hot cocoa drink, a bowl of berries with yoghurt, or some dark chocolate with a cup of tea. You could also try these other options (occasionally):

- 1 bag of popcorn.

- 1 mini bar (35g) of good quality dark chocolate (85 per cent cocoa solids).

- 1 small ice cream or ice lolly.

REMEMBER TO TAKE TIME OUT AND DO SOMETHING THAT IS NOT RELATED TO FOOD OR EXERCISE EACH WEEK.

For me, the priority was to sort out my food intake for match days, as well as the days before. From the plan above, we put together the ideal match-day menu:

BREAKFAST: Porridge with oat or almond milk (unsweetened) and berries. An hour later I would have a proper breakfast of a couple of eggs, half a slice of rye bread and half an avocado.

SNACK: Mid-morning, I would have half a pot of hummus or some cottage cheese as a snack.

LUNCH: Lunch would be grilled fish, with grilled veggies and sweet potato, brown rice or salad.

SNACK: In the afternoon, I'd have another snack – an apple, a spoonful of nut butter or a banana smoothie.

DINNER: At 6–7pm I'd have my evening meal – steak, salad and vegetables

I learned that on the day of a match I definitely shouldn't eat too much bulk – keeping my diet light but balanced with all food groups when I'm playing gives me energy for the whole day. Sweet potato is my new best friend. It keeps me full and I love the taste. It's a carb I really enjoy eating. Now the snacks I go for when I'm taking five at the side of the snooker table are prawns, beetroot, bean salads and smoothies.

"NOW THE SNACKS I GO FOR WHEN I'M TAKING FIVE AT THE SIDE OF THE SNOOKER TABLE ARE PRAWNS, BEETROOT, BEAN SALADS AND SMOOTHIES"

BRAIN GAINS

Before we started, it was important that I understood exactly which foods I really love to eat and the impact they would have on me. If I was going to change everything, I wanted to know exactly what benefits I'd see and how quickly I'd see them. For me, it was all about identifying my goals early on and knowing what I was working towards. I was looking forward to my brain feeling fully switched on again.

CARBS = GLUCOSE = BRAIN POWER

Rhiannon gave me a list of carbohydrates that contain lots of fibre and slow-releasing energy, and I began to incorporate them into my daily routine.

EXAMPLES OF MY GO-TO CARBOHYDRATES:

- Wholegrain bread

- Rye bread

- Oats

- Sweet potato

- Potato

- Rice

- Wholegrain rice

- Buckwheat

- Quinoa

I worked hard to make sure that my fat portions went back to a normal amount for one person – things like half an avocado each day, instead of two whole ones. These small steps ensured that I had a routine in place. Part of it was about realising that, just because something is technically good for you, it doesn't mean you have to eat all of it!

I had occasionally tried to fast in an attempt to lose weight, but the only affect of this was low energy and limited concentration levels, neither of which were ideal for someone who was paid to play snooker for hours on end. The first changes that we made to my diet were small and simple, but extremely effective.

Having breakfast every morning was essential. This meant that I exchanged egg white omelettes for a far superior and satisfying whole egg omelette, with vegetables and a slice of rye bread. Before I started on the plan, I thought I was eating way too much food, and that was why I was getting bigger. I realised that it was actually more a case of eating the wrong things and of erratic and unstructured eating. This is often called mindless eating, which basically means eating without really acknowledging what you are putting into your body, and why.

As a result of mindless eating, you end up finishing meals quickly and then eating more than your body needs. To help combat this, porridge, eggs and smoothies were all back on the menu, as were planned snacks, lunches and dinners, all of which were full of colour.

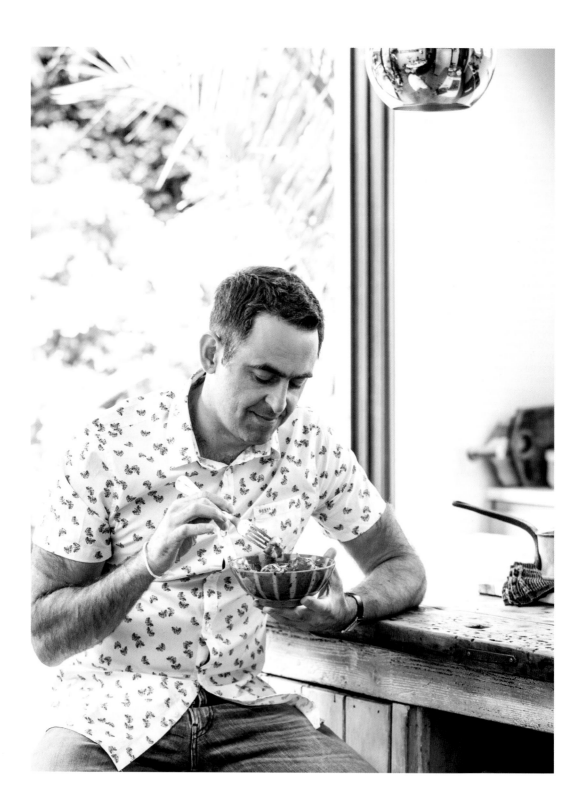

BRAIN GAIN RECIPES:

Breakfast Omelette

Cinnamon Spice Overnight Oats

Rainbow Chilli Stir Fry

Jacket Sweet Potato and Homemade Beans

Baked Salmon with Fresh Chilli and Ginger

Oat Smoothie

EATING FOR BODY

My way of living hasn't helped me over the years, especially when it came to my attitude to food and training. I was locked in a cycle in which I would over-eat, before punishing myself with exercise that pushed my body to the limit. It was destructive and counter-productive – we all know that hard training can only take you so far. In order to see the physical changes that we want to see when we start a new regime, we have to get our food intake right. If we don't, there's no chance of seeing as much improvement and we're more likely to give up and go back to our old ways.

I didn't cut myself any slack. If I went for a long run I would eat well, but on the days I didn't run, I'd eat badly. The same approach went for the biscuit jar or the chocolate bar: if I had one chocolate, the 'I've blown it' mindset would kick in; I'd feel like I'd 'failed' and a period of binge eating would begin, followed by a week of restrictive eating and another week of binge eating. Without realising it, I was trapped in the vicious circle of bingeing and then restricting. This mindset meant that I over-exercised and ran excessively nearly every single day, in order to compensate for eating badly.

Being stuck in this mentality also meant that my eating was chaos. I was over-exercising and following a high-fat, low-carb diet that was not fuelling my body efficiently for my mad workouts! What I was putting in was preventing the loss of body fat that I so badly wanted. Rhiannon basically told me that I was malnourished, which made no sense to me – I felt heavier than ever. But she explained that the injuries I kept on getting were from a lack of fuel and overtraining.

Fad diets might result in some weight loss for a short period of time at the start, but it's a world full of broken promises. It's not a sustainable way of eating – it often cuts whole food groups and the nutrition everyone needs to feel on top form. As I've already said, I needed carbohydrates in my diet but wasn't getting them, because I had decided that they made me fat. The actual reality was that my muscles were starved of fuel and my body wasn't performing well. After introducing a balanced list of foods, I began to exercise less, eat more of the right foods consistently and lose the body fat that I was so desperate to shift.

> WHEN I FIRST WENT INTO RHIANNON'S CLINIC, I WEIGHED 14 STONE 12LBS WITH A 34-INCH WAIST AND NOW I WEIGH 13 STONE 3LBS AND HAVE A 32-INCH WAIST.

EXTRA NUTRITION TO SUPPORT MY RUNNING

To get back to my running peak (which also helped my snooker), I needed to learn how to refuel properly to prevent injury and help keep my performance high. We discussed what types of food I should eat before and after a run to achieve maximum results. I also realised that I needed lots of different mind-and-body-friendly vitamins and minerals.

Vitamins are available in two forms: water-soluble and fat-soluble.

WATER-SOLUBLE VITAMINS are easily lost through bodily fluids and must be replaced each day – B vitamins and vitamin C, for example.

FAT-SOLUBLE VITAMINS tend to accumulate within the body and are not needed on a daily basis. The fat-soluble vitamins are A, D, E and K.

We've identified that mindset is the biggest key to success, but it generally comes really low down on our to-do list. For me, the key is working out what your goals are and having a champion's mind when it comes to achieving them. Anyone can go to the gym and wander about for an hour, lifting weights and hoping for the best, but it's all about making time for your fitness and making things consistent.

As Rhiannon taught me, it all starts with how you fuel your body: give it nothing and you will get nothing. Motivation, goal-setting, tracking your progress – these are all things to keep an eye on. But it all starts with what you eat.

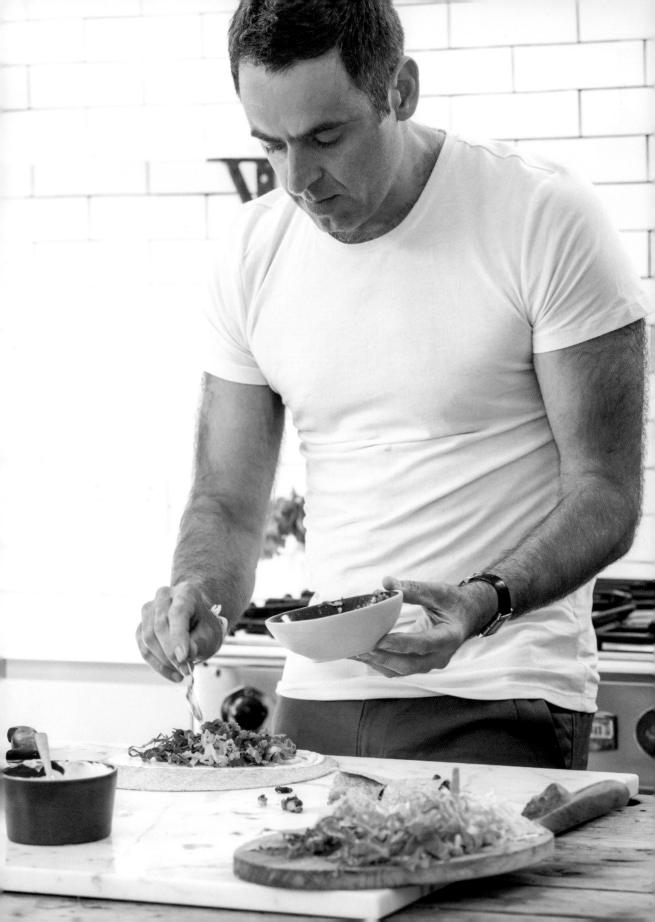

"NUTRIENT INTAKE BEFORE YOU START TRAINING WILL HELP MAXIMISE YOUR PERFORMANCE"

FOOD TO EAT BEFORE A RUN – CARBS, PROTEINS, VEG AND FATS

Complex carbohydrates 2–3 hours before a run.

Nutrient intake before you start training will help maximise your performance, in addition to making sure you don't damage your muscles.

If you plan on training within 2–3 hours of eating, you need a substantial amount of energy to keep you going before and during your workout.

Try opting for a healthy, balanced meal of carbohydrates, protein and fat such as:

- Scrambled eggs on wholegrain toast, with half an avocado.

- Chicken or salmon with quinoa and roasted vegetables.

Alternatively if you're on the go, make a smoothie from milk, banana, protein powder and oats to give you longer lasting energy.

Make sure you eat some easy-to-digest carbohydrates 1–2 hours before you plan to train.

If you are fuelling your workout 1–2 hours before it, you don't want to overdo it and feel too full to exercise, but you do need to ensure you've provided your body with enough energy to maximise your performance.

Try:

- Mixed fruit with Greek yoghurt and seeds.

- Banana with oatcakes and nut butter.

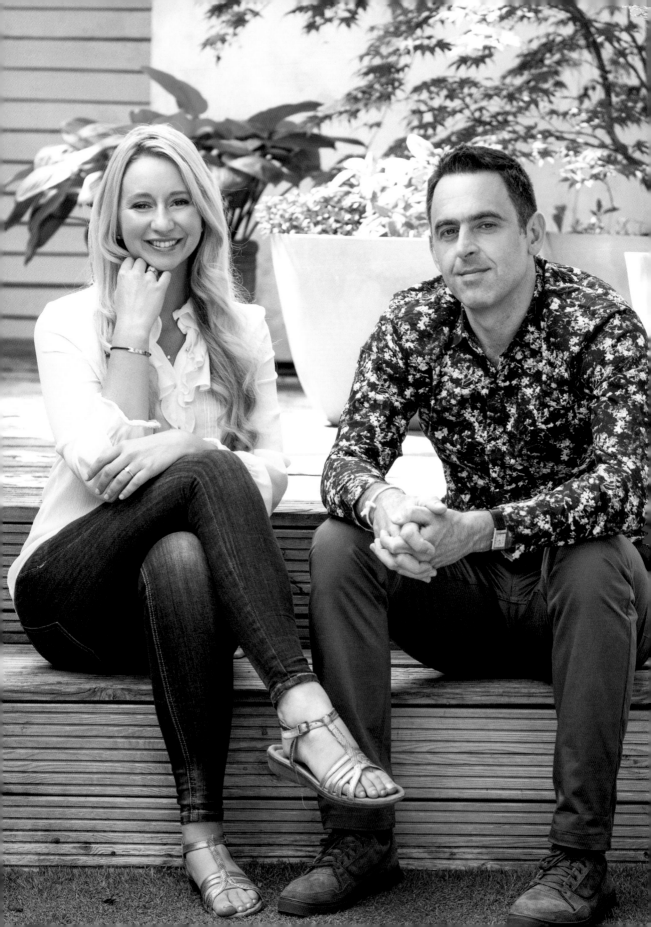

FOOD TO EAT AFTER A RUN

Having had more injuries than I would have liked during my career, I know that refuelling your body after a workout is really important in aiding muscle recovery. After exercising, your glycogen stores will be really low, so you need to refuel them.

The best foods to refuel:

- Chicken or turkey, with sweet potato and vegetables.

- Pasta, with salmon and roasted vegetables.

- Lentil, mixed bean and white rice salad, with avocado.

White carbs like rice are great post-workout foods because they can be accessed quickly by the body.

NUTRIENTS, NOT NUMBERS

The thing I worried about most when it came to getting healthy was that I'd have to start keeping a long list of everything I'd eaten. The idea of counting calories gets a big 'no' from me, partly because it can never be 100 per cent accurate.

A calorie is a unit of energy – the kilocalorie that is used to measure food energy is the amount of energy required to heat one kilogram of water by one degree Celsius. Food calorie counts come from chemical analysis into food's carbohydrate, fat and protein contents, which are then added together using the energy values for each nutrient.

While many people treat calorie estimates as concrete figures, they are only approximations and don't take into account individual differences in food absorption, metabolism, or the effect of cooking a food on our ability to digest it.

And we also need to remember the hidden stuff. Food companies do not add sugar, fat and salt to their products for fun; they do it because we like them and, once we start eating them, we want more. To put it simply, calories taste good and can pop up where we least expect them. Manufacturers have spent millions of pounds trying to make low-calorie food taste as good as high-calorie food, but to most people's taste buds, they've failed. Let's face it; we still reach for the biscuit tin when we want a treat.

And don't forget that a number cannot dictate how healthy something is for you; after all, 100 calories of broccoli and 100 calories of chocolate will provide the body with very different nutrients.

THE BLOOD SUGAR ROLLERCOASTER

Many of us get stuck on what I call a 'blood sugar rollercoaster', meaning that we end up in a vicious circle of wanting high-sugar foods and relying on fast-releasing energy to keep us going throughout the day. These cravings have nothing to do with willpower, but are a result of the reaction that happens when our bodies respond to foods that are high in sugar. They make everything go up and down, including our ability to concentrate; before you know it, you're going around in a circle, sabotaging your food choices and heading for the items that can provide you with that quick sugar fix.

Maintaining a steady blood sugar level throughout the day is important for helping your mood, energy and motivation. When your blood sugar is suddenly high, it will later 'crash' back down, meaning that you'll have mood swings and low energy levels.

Your blood sugar level depends on the carbohydrates and sugars that you eat. Simple carbohydrates have often been stripped of their nutritional value by the time they make it to your plate. These include refined grains and added sugars, which are found in foods like white bread, cakes, pre-packaged goods, sweets and fizzy drinks. These are known as fast-releasing sugars and they can get into your system very quickly, which is what causes the blood sugar 'spike'. These carbs are not bad for us but they aren't the best choice for eating regularly. Complex carbohydrates such as whole grains, brown rice, oats and quinoa are known as slow-releasing carbohydrates, as they are an excellent source of fibre. Fibre slows down the release of the energy contained in the food, which means that they give you more energy, for longer. Fruit is also packed with fibre, which slows down the release of the sugars from the fruit, meaning it does not spike your blood sugar.

When you eat carbohydrates, your body begins to digest them and change them into glucose, which is then sent to the blood stream. The conversion to glucose happens to all carbohydrates but the difference between sugars, refined grains and complex carbohydrates is how long they take to convert. I started to learn that food with lots of fibre is the best thing for someone like me, who has to concentrate for hours on end and who needs to stay calm and steady – feeling my energy levels crashing is just about the worst thing that can happen when I'm competing or watching others play!

Rhiannon taught me that foods that are high in fibre take longer to digest, which obviously gives us lasting energy that is released into our system throughout the day. On the other hand, simple sugars and refined grains are broken down and converted into glucose extremely quickly, which means our blood glucose levels will experience the 'spike', resulting in instant energy that can sometimes make you feel 'hyper' if you don't have enough of the other fibre items in your meal. But this does not last for very long and you will soon find yourself craving that sugar rush again.

> **SYMPTOMS OF LOW BLOOD SUGAR INCLUDE: FATIGUE, MOOD SWINGS, IRRITABILITY, ANXIETY, DEPRESSIVE SYMPTOMS.**

The reason why low blood sugar may result in such extreme symptoms is because glucose is the only thing that fuels our brain. So if you are depriving your brain of its only fuel, you are practically starving it, meaning it will begin to malfunction. This explained a lot about my performance and also my mood.

So how can we prevent ourselves from becoming victims of this cycle that leads us to crave sugar? The answer is simple: we should add more fibre to our diet and opt for whole grains where possible. Try to include more of the starchy carbohydrates that are high in fibre, such as wholegrain rice, pasta, bread, potatoes, quinoa, beans and lentils, and eat fewer of the high-sugar varieties. By adding more fruits, vegetables and whole grains to your plate, you are effectively adding more vitamins and minerals to your diet and helping to stabilise your blood sugar levels. This will help you focus, think more clearly and regulate your mood.

"MAINTAINING A STEADY BLOOD SUGAR LEVEL THROUGHOUT THE DAY IS IMPORTANT FOR HELPING YOUR MOOD"

BACK TO BASICS NUTRITION

CARBOHYDRATES

Carbohydrates hold a special place in nutrition, as they provide the largest single source of energy in the diet. Most of them get broken down or transformed into glucose, which can be used as energy. They can also be turned into fat, which is energy that is stored for later use. Glucose is the essential fuel for our brains and the energy source that our muscles prefer during strenuous exercise.

If you've ever been on a strict dietary regime avoiding carbohydrates, you'll know that it can be hard to concentrate and that you often experience severe mood swings –this is because carbohydrates play an important role in creating serotonin (the happy hormone) in the brain.

No matter what sport you enjoy, whether it be running, swimming, tennis or snooker, carbohydrates are essential for maximising performance. The amount of carbohydrate your muscles will need for energy will depend on your training programme, as well as your dietary goals. Generally, the more full-on your workout is, the more energy you will need; not fuelling the body with the right amount of energy may lead to early fatigue, loss of concentration and achy muscles. Ultimately, performance and recovery can be maximised and supported by sufficient amounts of carbohydrates, as it is stored in the muscles as glycogen. However, these stores are limited and need to be 'topped up' regularly, in order to support regular activity.

COMPLEX CARBOHYDRATES

WHOLEGRAIN BREAD

QUINOA

BROWN RICE

BUCKWHEAT

STARCHY VEGETABLES

OATS

FRUITS

LEGUMES

There is definitely a case for reducing refined carbohydrates (the least nutritious type – things like white bread and white pasta). You should instead opt for complex carbohydrates, as they release their energy more slowly. Think about 'grains' rather than 'carbs' – it's simpler to understand and remember.

OTHER CARBOHYDRATES

SUGARY DRINKS: Artificially sweetened drinks are some of the unhealthiest things you can put into your body.

FRUIT JUICES: These may have similar effects to sugar-sweetened beverages, as they lack the natural fibre that the fruit contains.

WHITE BREAD: These refined carbohydrates are often low in essential nutrients when not fortified.

PASTRIES: These refined carbohydrates tend to be very high in sugar.

ICE CREAM: Most types are very high in sugar.

CHOCOLATE: Obviously high in sugar, but you should opt for good-quality dark chocolate (70 per cent-plus cocoa solids) as a less unhealthy option.

FRENCH FRIES AND CRISPS: Whole potatoes are healthy, but once they are deep-fried they are not. These foods may be fine in moderation for some, but many of us should limit how many of them we eat.

Those who advocate a low-carb diet often claim that carbohydrates are not essential nutrients in the diet. It's true that the body can function without a single gram of carbohydrate in the diet, but just because they are not essential for survival, that doesn't mean they aren't beneficial. The bottom line is that carbohydrates in their natural, fibre-rich form are healthy.

There is no one-size-fits-all solution to nutrition. Your optimal carbohydrate intake will depend on numerous factors, such as age, gender, metabolic health and physical activity. If you are looking to lose weight or if you have health problems like metabolic syndrome or type 2 diabetes, you are more likely to be carbohydrate-sensitive, in which case, reducing carbohydrate intake can have clear benefits. On the other hand, if you're a healthy person who is just trying to stay healthy, there is probably no reason for you to avoid carbohydrates. And if you are naturally lean and physically active, then you may even function much better with plenty of them in your diet.

PROTEIN

It's really important to make sure you have protein throughout the day because when you smash the exercise you are effectively breaking down your muscles. That's why so many gyms sell protein bars and we are used to seeing people drinking their shakes after a big workout — it basically helps to increase the impact of exercise.

If you eat protein before a workout, you give your body the amino acids that help to prevent muscle breakdown. While athletes might need more protein than the average person, one of the biggest myths regarding their intake is that eating large amounts will result in huge muscles. Athletes who strength train require an increased protein intake (1.2–1.7g per kg of body-weight per day) as do endurance athletes (1.2–1.4g per kg of body-weight per day) compared to the average person who should consume 0.8–1.0g per kg of body-weight per day. If our desired energy requirements are being met, a well-balanced diet will contain enough protein to meet any increased requirements. Research has suggested that an additional 15–25g of protein can have a number of benefits in a post-workout meal: these include boosting glycogen storage, reducing muscle soreness and promoting muscle recovery, but all this depends on how you are working out and how much protein you have in your normal diet.

The best tip to obtain results more quickly is to break up the protein you eat throughout the day. Grazing on it, rather than packing it all into one big meal, will significantly boost protein synthesis, which is required for muscles growth and a necessary process for maintaining strength. However, research suggests that a healthy, balanced diet can provide the protein needed for muscle recovery, so you don't need to worry about expensive powders and supplements. If you eat right, the old-fashioned way should be enough.

FAT

Fats are the most energy-dense of all the macronutrients and are essential for healthy living. There are many different types of fat, and when you're doing a good workout, they play a big part in accessing the body's stored carbohydrate. Basically, the body needs to break the fat down and transport it to the muscles, so it can be used as energy and boost your workout.

Learning all this from Rhiannon blew my mind – I had to get my head around the fact that fat was not only good for you, but also that it could help sustain energy levels throughout the day. Fat takes longer to break down into energy that the body can use, and this is why your body uses it when it is resting. Adding in 'good' fats to your diet, in addition to eating fewer refined carbohydrates, will help your body step up its ability to burn fat for energy.

FOOD FOR PERFORMANCE:

MONOUNSATURATED AND OMEGA-3 FATS. THE BEST SOURCES OF THESE TYPES OF FAT COME FROM OLIVE OIL, AVOCADOS, NUTS, SEEDS AND OILY FISH.

I couldn't understand why you would want to eat fat if you were trying to eat healthily. I soon realised that if you show your body that it is getting a consistent source of fat from your diet, it will be more likely to let go of the fat it is currently holding. Fat is energy, and your body does not want to give up this invaluable source of fuel – we may think fat's a total pain, but your body thinks otherwise.

HYDRATE

Our bodies are made largely of water, so it's understandable that every function inside them depends on it to do its job. Cells, organs and tissue all need water, so it's essential that we drink up. When we have enough water we become more efficient at losing it, through sweating and urination. The amount of sweating I used to do was criminal, and the idea that I needed to be taking in more water felt like a joke! But I soon realised that drinking more water would help regulate everything. The more water I drank, the more relaxed my body was.

Use this equation to find out your ideal daily water intake:

TAKE YOUR WEIGHT (KG) AND DIVIDE BY 30 =
THE AMOUNT OF WATER YOU NEED (LITRES)

Good hydration has been shown to enhance and keep performance steady, which is what I was lacking, while dehydration has been linked to poor performance, weakness and fatigue. Who knew a simple bottle of water could have such a big impact!

In this section I've tried to help you get your head around the basics. I also hope that showing you where I was will help you to see that whatever your situation, there are things you can do to get yourself back on track. There's no doubt that I'd lost my way, and sitting down with Rhiannon to understand why I ate like I did was an important first step. The next move was to look at how I could sort myself out, and that came with looking at what I put on my plate.

WHAT IS ON YOUR PLATE?

PLATES – WHAT SHOULD BE ON YOURS?

We eat for many different reasons and it would be impossible to cover them all. But in this section, I want to think about how we decide what to eat, and what we want from it. Obviously the first answer is that we eat to not feel hungry, but for me, eating tends to be either about helping myself to perform to the best standard or about helping a particular bit of the body that I know needs a bit of TLC. In this section, I want to show what you can achieve if you put a bit of thought into your meals.

EXAMPLES OF MY PLATES:

MOOD OR MENTAL HEALTH PLATE

ON THE ROAD OR EATING OUT PLATE

GUT PLATE

FITNESS OR TRAINING DAY PLATE

PRE-TOURNAMENT OR
TRAINING PLATE

FUELLING FITNESS

EATING HEALTHILY TRUMPS EXERCISE, PURE AND SIMPLE. When food and fitness combine well together, that's the best scenario. The problem is that when you rely on exercise alone, it often comes back to bite you. This is partly because of appetite hormones, which make you feel like you are starving after exercise – this is why, no matter how much I was running, the weight just wasn't shifting. I would do lots of exercise, and even though I was trying to be good with what I ate, I found myself eating too much of the bad stuff.

What I came to realise was that if my food was good, I could train better and see more obvious results. Doing this also meant that my head was clearer and allowed me to nail my snooker.

I used to like working out every day to keep my head clear, but I now know that it was excessive, and so I need a routine that allows for rest days (which are essential for body toning, muscle repair and improving muscle definition) and is manageable around my snooker.

MY ADVICE: BE SENSIBLE WITH YOUR GOALS FOR INDIVIDUAL SESSIONS. ATTEMPTING A 15-MILE RUN IN YOUR FIRST WEEK IS PROBABLY NOT THAT CLEVER! BUT MIXING IT UP WITH 20 MINUTES OF MODERATE INTENSITY EXERCISE (LIKE RIDING A BIKE AND 30 MINUTES OF LOW INTENSITY EXERCISE LIKE WALKING OR SWIMMING) WILL MEAN YOU SEE RESULTS.

TIPS:

1. **MIX IT UP.** Eat a varied and balanced diet that provides your body with the right amount of energy and essential nutrients.

2. **FUEL RIGHT.** Eat a variety of foods. including some that contain carbohydrates, based on the amount of exercise you want to achieve.

3. **STRIVE FOR FIVE.** Eat at least five portions of fruit and vegetables a day; fresh, frozen, dried and canned all count.

4. **REFUEL**. If you need to recover quickly, start refuelling with carbohydrate foods and fluids as soon as possible after exercise.

5. **THINK FLUID.** Ensure you are well-hydrated by drinking throughout the day, as well as before, during and after exercise.

Sitting down and looking at my diet was the best thing I ever did, and it also made me examine my daily routine. Once I got into the rhythm of eating on schedule, it was time to look at how I exercised physically and mentally, and bring it all together.

"SITTING DOWN AND LOOKING AT MY DIET WAS THE BEST THING I EVER DID"

MY TRAINING SCHEDULE

I get up at 7am and drink a cup of herbal tea and a glass of water, and then eat half a slice of rye bread with nut butter. Once I've fuelled up, I'll head out for 30 minutes on a steady 4-mile run. When I hit a 7-minute mile, my heart rate will average at 160, which is steady state training, good for keeping a strong fitness base.

After my run, I'll do four to eight strides of around 60–100 metres, which means running at around 90 per cent effort and achieving a 5-minute mile pace. I do this so I can keep the speed in my legs, which sets me up for my next run or training session the next day. Once I'm back from the run, I'll stretch and loosen up.

On another day I'll do the same thing, but then I'll go to the boxing gym and do some pad work or will spar with some other boxers non-stop for 20–30 minutes. This will be a heavier workout, but it's good because it incorporates cross-training and also complements my running.

I'll sometimes do other types of running: I'll warm up for 5–10 minutes and then find a hill with a steady incline and do 8–12 repetitions of between 30 and 60 seconds, all depending on what I'm trying to achieve.

Once I'm back home, I'll shower and eat a breakfast of porridge followed by egg and avocado.

FITTING IN A WORKOUT

For me, exercise has to easily fit into my day and I have to be able to mix it up a bit. You aren't going to stick to anything that you don't like, so the key is to make it as enjoyable as possible.

As I am often away playing, I can't always get to the gym and do the workout I want, so I have to make the best of what I have. My main aim is to get my heart rate up, that's when you know you are doing your best work. Sometimes if time is short and I am in a hotel room, I do my stairs workout, which involves going up 10 flights of stairs, getting the lift back down, and going again as many times as I can. It's simple but very effective.

My other travelling workout includes:

Weights	Gilder shoulders
Press ups	Burpees
Squats	Star jumps, chest out.
Chest press	

If I can get to the gym, I like to give myself a proper challenge, so I throw together lots of different exercises and see how far I can push it. My own workout can be any number of the following exercises. You don't have to do loads, getting through just a few exercises is better than not doing any.

My classic go-to exercises that can make up any workout are:

Burpees	Lunges
Press ups	Sit ups, vi-sits
Narrow press ups	High knees
Sit ups	Plank

When you have more time and are in your routine, another good way to get fit is to take up a sport: boxing, football, badminton, dancing, running. Find a local club that does these activities and just have a go. Sometimes doing something you enjoy is motivating; you'll go more often if you're having fun and, more importantly, you'll stick with it in the long-term. You can meet good friends, too – you'll be surprised how enjoyable it can be! A great class or team run definitely beats the gym for me.

BRAIN HEALTH ON A PLATE

We all know it isn't easy to eat 'well' all the time, but when we crave the bad stuff, it's usually our body telling us that it needs a well-balanced meal with plenty of nutrients. In order to prepare the best food for the mind, we should consider the foods that help with positive brain function and mood enhancement. If you put all the food groups below on a plate, you'll be pretty much there.

Rather than counting calories or macronutrients, Rhiannon encouraged me to use my hands to roughly estimate portion sizes. You only need to be careful about measuring your portion size in the first week. After that, you'll get an eye for it and it won't matter if your portions are a little over from time to time.

1 OUTSTRETCHED PALMFUL OF PROTEIN
– for example, chicken, fish or tofu

1 HANDFUL OF CARBOHYDRATES
– for example, oats, rice or starchy fruit and vegetables

2 HANDFULS OF NON-STARCHY VEGETABLES
– for example, broccoli, spinach or peppers

1 THUMB OF HEALTHY FATS
– for example, olive oil, butter, coconut oil or nut butter

HOW THIS WORKS:

CHICKEN: Chicken is a great source of lean protein, as well as being rich in other essential nutrients. It contains magnesium, phosphorus, potassium and zinc, and is also a good source of vitamins A, B6, B12, D, E and K. All these vitamins and minerals assist in maintaining a healthy immune system, regulating digestion and providing the body with energy.

BAKED SWEET POTATO: High in vitamin A, sweet potatoes are as delicious as they are nutritious. They are a great source of complex carbohydrates, which provide slow-release energy, and are also rich in fibre. Combining carbohydrates and protein also helps boost your serotonin production, which is our feel-good hormone.

OLIVE OIL: The fatty acid in olive oil is a monounsaturated fat called oleic acid, which has been linked with a variety of health benefits. There is a suggestion that it reduces inflammation, reduces the risk of neurodegenerative diseases such as Alzheimer's and also has beneficial effects on genes that are linked to cancer. The monounsaturated fats in olive oil are also fairly resistant to high heat, meaning that you don't risk losing its nutritional value if you choose to cook with it.

SESAME SEEDS: Seeds are a good source of the essential omega-3 fatty acid, which is extremely important for optimum brain function. Omega-3 intake has been linked to lessening depressive feelings. Seeds are also a great source of zinc – acute depletion of it may cause loss of taste and appetite, and it has also been linked to male reproductive health.

ROASTED VEGETABLES: I think adding as much colour as possible to your plate is the key – I've discovered that the more variety you have on your plate, the more micronutrients there are that benefit your gut. The gut has been named our 'second brain', which indicates that if your gut bacteria are diverse and healthy, then your brain will be too.

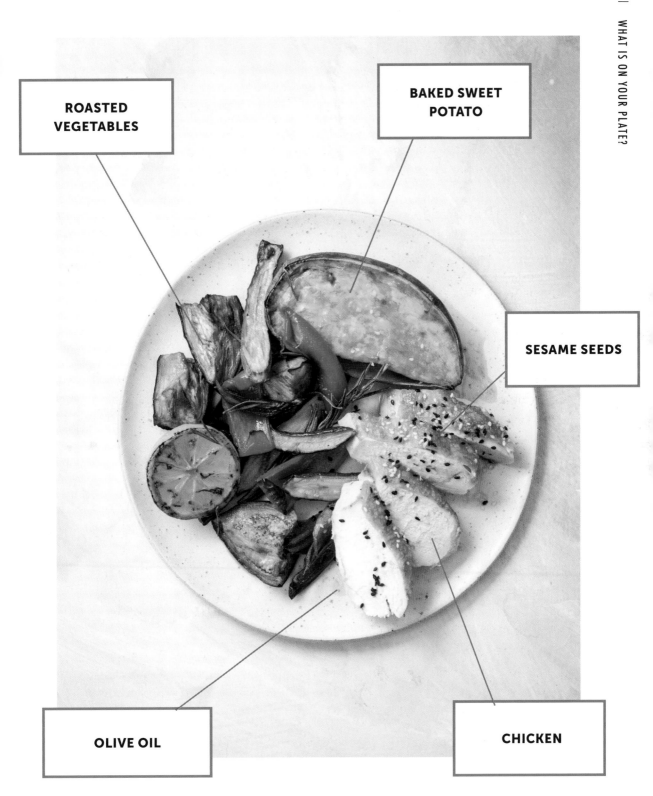

ROASTED VEGETABLES

BAKED SWEET POTATO

SESAME SEEDS

OLIVE OIL

CHICKEN

ON THE ROAD PLATE

It's easy to fall off the healthy-eating wagon in the early days of a new diet. There's also the big question: is it harder to stay focused when you are out and about and not cooking in your own kitchen? Lots of people find the first few weeks of a new diet easier if they stay at home and only eat meals that they've planned in advance. I know this is a way I can keep myself on track but I also know that it doesn't always work, especially when I'm competing, travelling and living out of hotel rooms. It's all about making sure you have delicious stuff on the go – it helps you steer clear of those old habits!

HUMMUS

Hummus is a big winner for me — it's my go-to snack, wherever I am. A small pot of it or a dollop in a lunch box is the ideal way to add some tasty good fats to your meal, not to mention some extra fibre and protein.

SERVES 4

4 tbsp olive oil, plus extra to serve

1 x 400g tin chickpeas, drained and rinsed

3 tbsp tahini

2 tbsp lemon juice

3 garlic cloves, very finely chopped

pinch of salt and black pepper

1. Blitz the chickpeas, tahini, lemon juice, garlic, salt and pepper, until it all starts to break down, then gradually pour in the remaining 4 tablespoons of olive oil with the motor still running.

FALAFEL

Falafel travels well, unlike meat and fish, which should be kept refrigerated. They can be eaten hot or cold and are a great source of protein. Most supermarkets sell mini pots of them and they come in many different varieties.

MAKES 8 PATTIES

1 x 400g tin of black beans

1 x 400g tin of chickpeas

1 lemon

1 tbsp tahini

1 tsp paprika

2 tbsp plain flour

1 bunch of fresh coriander

1 tbsp olive oil

1. Drain the beans and chickpeas, and blitz them in a food processor with all the ingredients apart from olive oil, until smooth.

2. Scrape out the mixture and use wet hands to divide and shape it into 8 patties about 1.5cm thick.

3. Heat a tablespoon of olive oil in a frying pan and add the falafels, turning when golden and crisp.

RICE SALAD: Add some sweetcorn and a basic lettuce, tomato and cucumber salad to some cold cooked rice. You can buy rice salad pots at most supermarkets, but making your own is a guaranteed way to get your perfect portion size and also lets you add some extras from the cupboard. Drizzle with olive oil and lemon juice, and a pinch of salt.

VEGETABLE STICKS: Make sticks of peppers, cucumber, carrots and celery to have with your dip or salad. If you like your vegetables roasted, then you can make some in advance to take with you, but you will also find bags of them readily available in many supermarkets.

FRUIT SALAD: It's always a good idea to get as much nutrition as possible when you are on the road. By adding a fruit salad to a yoghurt for dessert, you are increasing your micronutrient intake and also working towards your five a day!

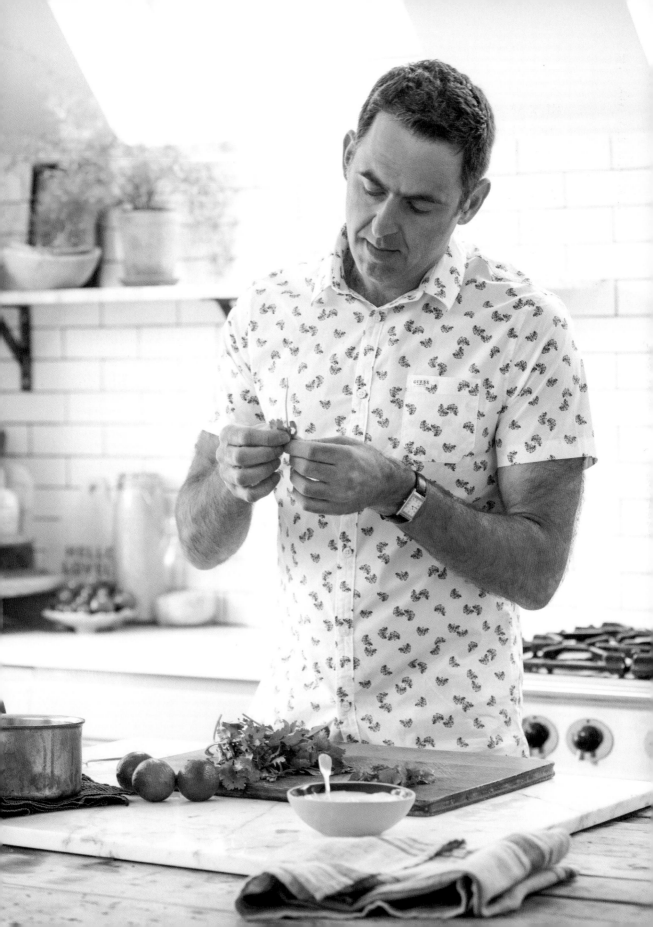

GUT HEALTH PLATE

I've had my fair share of stress, which often left my digestive system all over the place. The first step to a healthy diet is to make sure the digestion system is working properly – it's important that it is making proper use of all the nutrition you are putting into your body.

MACKEREL OR SALMON – Eating at least two portions of fish every week, including one of oily fish, will help to keep your blood pressure healthy and improve your blood lipid levels, both of which will reduce your risk of cardiovascular disease.

Rhiannon gave me a list of gut-friendly ingredients. I don't mind experimenting with different flavours and spices, so we developed the recipe opposite.

MISO AUBERGINE

Miso is a traditional Japanese seasoning produced by fermenting soy beans. Fermented foods are often linked to good gut health. Miso paste can be added to soups and salad dressings, or turned into a healthy mustard 'miso-mayo'. Use it to coat your aubergine before you roast it in the oven in the below recipe.

SERVES 2

2 large aubergines
3 tbsp olive oil

For the paste:
4 tbsp brown miso
3 tbsp honey
2 tbsp soy sauce
3 tbsp mirin
2 tsp sesame oil

To serve
Toasted sesame seeds
Spring onions, sliced

1. Turn the grill to a high heat. Halve 2 large aubergines lengthways and score the flesh in a criss-cross pattern.

2. Heat the olive oil in a frying pan and fry the aubergines, flesh side down, for 5 minutes, then flip and cook for 5 more minutes.

3. Mix the paste ingredients together in a bowl.

4. Put the aubergines on a baking tray and spread the paste on the flesh. Grill for around 4–5 minutes, before sprinkling with toasted sesame seeds and sliced spring onions to serve.

FISH FILLET: Wrap in baking paper and bake in the oven for 15 minutes until cooked.

SAUERKRAUT SALAD: Add sauerkraut to your daily salad for a tangy twist! The beneficial probiotics found in it are important for good digestive health. While more research is needed into the exact types of beneficial bacteria that are found in sauerkraut and other fermented foods, we do know that they 'feed' the good bacteria in your gut and can help to combat inflammation.

WHOLEGRAIN RICE: a serving of rice would go nicely with your aubergine and sauerkraut, and will deliver a lot of fibre, which promotes a healthy digestive tract.

MY TOP 5 BACTERIA-FRIENDLY (PROBIOTIC) FOODS

KEFIR: Kefir is a fermented probiotic milk drink that is made by adding kefir grains to cow's or goat's milk. Kefir grains are not cereal grains, but rather cultures of lactic acid bacteria and yeast. Kefir contains several major strains of 'friendly bacteria' and yeast, and like yoghurt, it is generally tolerated by people who are lactose intolerant.

SAUERKRAUT: Sauerkraut is finely shredded cabbage that has been fermented by lactic acid bacteria. In addition to its probiotic qualities, sauerkraut is rich in fibre, as well as vitamins B, C and K. It is also high in sodium and contains iron and manganese, as well as the antioxidants that are important for eye health. Always choose unpasteurised sauerkraut, as pasteurisation kills the live and active bacteria. A very traditional food, it is popular in many European countries.

YOGHURT: Yoghurt is made from milk that has been fermented by friendly bacteria. It can be better than milk for people with a lactose intolerance, because the bacteria turn some of the lactose into lactic acid, which is what gives it its sour taste. However, not all yoghurt contains live probiotics – in some cases they are killed during processing. Choose yoghurt with active or live cultures and always read the label, because many low-fat or fat-free yoghurts are often full of sugar.

KIMCHI: Kimchi is a fermented and spicy side dish that is popular in Korea. Cabbage is usually the main ingredient, but it can also be made from other vegetables. It contains lactic acid bacteria, including lactobacillus kimchii. Kimchi made from cabbage is high in vitamins and minerals, including vitamin K, riboflavin (vitamin B2) and iron.

KOMBUCHA: Kombucha is a tea drink fermented by a friendly bacteria and yeast. It is consumed in many parts of the world, and especially in Asia. There are many claims that it is good for health, though high-quality evidence is lacking. However, as it is fermented with bacteria and yeast, it is likely to have health benefits as a result of its probiotic properties.

MISCONCEPTIONS AROUND GUT HEALTH

Much of the information surrounding gut health is confusing and hard to understand. Before I began to learn about food, I didn't have any idea that the gut was so complicated and that it has such a big effect on how we feel – it definitely affected my mood and energy levels. Here are some of the most frequent misconceptions of gut health, as well as some clarifications.

GLUTEN

There has been a lot of discussion about gluten being 'bad' for our gut health. Gluten is a protein that is found in most grains, including wheat, barley, rye and oats. It has been portrayed as a big problem, due to the misconception that carbohydrates make you fat. Many people have also started self-diagnosing themselves with a gluten intolerance. This has led to a rise in products that are free from gluten, though many gluten-free products are high in sugar and contain less nutrients, due to lower levels of fibre and fat.

But the reality is that research shows that only 1–7 per cent of the population are actually affected by non-coeliac gluten sensitivity, and only 1–2 per cent are diagnosed with coeliac disease. Coeliac disease requires the strict avoidance of gluten in any food, and even cross-contamination can cause gut problems. Non-coeliac gluten sensitivity means small amounts are often acceptable.

"CONSUMING VEGETABLES IS ONE OF THE BEST WAYS TO IMPROVE YOUR GUT HEALTH"

In truth, our bodies benefit from whole grains – they aid brain functioning, give us energy and improve gut health. Therefore, you shouldn't avoid foods that contain gluten, unless you really need to.

CHARCOAL

It might sound strange, but charcoal is another supplement that has gained a lot of attention recently, though there's not actually any evidence that it benefits us. While it's said to absorb the toxins in the gut, it could also be absorbing all the good nutrients we want our bodies to have.

FRUIT AND VEGETABLES

We need to eat fruit and vegetables on a daily basis and consuming a variety of them is key, as each one contains different nutrients. Consuming vegetables is one of the best ways to improve your gut health; rather than taking a probiotic supplement, save your money and stock your fridge with fruit and vegetables. Dietary fibre can be found in nuts, legumes, fruit and vegetables. Try increasing your intake of onions, garlic, chicory and figs to aid gut health. I'm not telling you to become vegetarian or vegan, but introducing more vegetables can increase your nutrient intake and make your gut healthier. Why not try meat-free Monday and see how your gut feels?

FITNESS PLATE

PORRIDGE, WALNUTS, BERRIES, ALMOND MILK AND FLAXSEED

This is my go-to plate after a run, when I need to re-fuel my body.

SERVES 1

50g rolled oats (or use
   jumbo oats)

40g berries of your choice

1 banana, thinly sliced

250ml milk of your choice
   (I like almond milk)

1 tsp ground cinnamon

A handful of chopped
   walnuts

A sprinkle of flaxseed

1. Put the oats, half of the sliced banana and the milk in a small pan. Cook over a medium heat for 3–5 minutes until the porridge is creamy and has thickened, stirring regularly.

2. Transfer to a bowl and top with the rest of the banana, the berries, the nuts and sprinkle with the cinnamon.

"IF YOU NEED TO RECOVER QUICKLY, START REFUELLING WITH CARBOHYDRATE FOODS AND FLUIDS AS SOON AS POSSIBLE AFTER EXERCISE"

PRE-TOURNAMENT PLATE

ROASTED FISH WITH BAKED SWEET POTATO

What I eat before a match has undergone the biggest transformation since I began my new nutrition plan. I think about what I need in a totally different way now, and it means that I approach matches with a calm focus and a clear head. My favourite dish to eat before a match is fish with roasted vegetables, green salad with avocado and a baked sweet potato.

For the fish

1 fillet of sea bass
   (or cod or haddock)

1 tsp olive oil

A pinch of salt

1 tsp mixed herbs

For the roasted vegetables

1 red pepper

1 red onion

½ aubergine

1 courgette

80g carrots

80g cherry tomatoes

1 tsp paprika

For the sweet potato

1 sweet potato

1 tsp butter (optional)

To serve

1 bag of mixed salad
   leaves

½ avocado

1 tbsp balsamic vinegar

A lemon wedge

1 tbsp olive oil

A pinch of salt

1. Pre-heat the oven to 180°C/Fan 160°C/Gas Mark 4.

2. Pierce the potato and put it in the oven for 50 minutes.

3. Chop the vegetables into small chunks and spread them evenly on a baking tray.

4. Drizzle with olive oil and sprinkle with paprika, before placing in the oven for 40 minutes.

5. Meanwhile, prepare your green salad. Add the leaves, avocado, salt, olive oil and a squeeze of lemon juice to a large bowl and mix well. Top with balsamic vinegar.

6. When there is 10 minutes of cooking time for the roasted vegetables remaining, heat the olive oil in a non-stick frying pan.

7. Once the pan is hot, season the fish with salt and place in the pan skin-side down, pressing down on the fillets to ensure the skin cooks evenly.

8. Cook for 3–4 minutes, until the skin is golden, and then carefully turn the fish over and cook for another minute. When the flesh is opaque, the fish is cooked.

9. Remove the potato from the oven. Slice it in half, and serve with a small amount of butter, some roasted vegetables and your salad.

10. Don't forget that leftover roasted vegetables will keep in an airtight container for the next day!

MINDFUL EATING

Eating can also have an effect on the gut. Our brain is directly connected to our thoughts, and a happy mind typically means a happy gut. In order to eat mindfully, try to focus on what you are doing and avoid distractions, whether that's the television or your phone. Instead, just focus on the food you are eating, what it is giving you and what it tastes like. By introducing this sort of mindful eating you will not only find that you enjoy your food more, but also that your gut will be able to digest the food more easily, making you feel healthier and happier all round.

This was one of the things I tried to do right at the start, and it took a lot of practice! Part of my problem was that, before, I'd just load up my plate and eat at 100 miles an hour. I never thought about what I needed to play my best snooker or to feel the best I could. I didn't ever think about what food would keep me going and release its energy slowly to help me focus. I didn't understand why I needed to make better choices, so just ate what was put in front of me, or what came around on the trolley before and during matches – there's not a lot that's healthy on there, believe me!

Rhiannon taught me that digestion is a very complex thing and involves a series of hormonal signals that work across the gut and our nervous system. Most evidence suggests that it takes around 20 minutes for the brain to acknowledge when we are feeling full, which explains why when someone eats too quickly, they can carry on eating a lot more. That was definitely me!

She also explained that research is increasingly recommending mindful eating, and that slower and more thoughtful eating can help with weight problems. This idea is based on the Buddhist approach to mindfulness, which involves being fully aware of what is happening within and around you. Similar techniques have even been used to help relieve stress and sort out problems like high blood pressure and chronic gastrointestinal difficulties.

Here are a few examples of things you can do to get started and to be more engaged when you eat:

- Acknowledge colours, flavours, textures and smells.

- Chew food slowly.

- Lose the TV or mobile phone at mealtimes.

- Learn skills to cope with anxiety and guilt around food.

- Make realistic goals.

- Mindfully sit down for meals, and try making an effort to plate or present your food differently.

- Chew your food for 30 seconds on the first bite, thinking about its texture and taste.

- Keep kitchen counters clear of all foods, apart from healthy ones.

- Avoid eating directly from a packet, and always pre-portion food.

- Eat something hot within the first hour of waking up.

- Avoid going more than 3–4 hours without eating anything.

- Put down your knife and fork between bites, to help slow down your eating.

STAYING ON TOP OF YOUR GAME.

CHANGE YOUR ATTITUDE AND CHANGE YOUR BODY:
WHAT I KNOW NOW

THE RUNNING WAS SOMETHING THAT I'D HID BEHIND, but once I got my head around the fact that good health is 80 per cent diet, it was like a light bulb moment. The main thing was realising that, even if I have the odd slip up, I can nip it in the bud the next day. Before, a bad day would become a bad month, but now I can have a little bit of bread and butter pudding and stop, without eating two!

IT WAS GREAT THAT RESULTS OF MY NEW REGIME HAPPENED QUICKLY, because if the penny doesn't drop immediately with me, I find it hard to stick to anything – I'd prefer to do something my way, until you can convince me that your way is the right way!

A HEALTHY DIET IS ALL ABOUT WHAT YOU EAT, the amount of it you eat and how many times a week you eat it.

SUGAR IS BEST IN SMALL AMOUNTS; I have cut down on it and now opt for unsweetened and fortified versions of the sweet plant-based milks I used to drink – lots of them contain added sugar, and I had no idea!

'HEALTHY' OPTIONS CAN BE COMPLETELY DECEPTIVE. I was eating two avocados every day, but I ended up losing my mind as I wasn't getting any carbohydrates to feed my brain. Imagine trying to be a professional snooker player who can't concentrate!

I THINK MY RELATIONSHIP WITH FOOD HAS PROBABLY ALWAYS BEEN ABOUT INDULGENCE and something I used to fix my 'snooker depression'. I love what I do, but the game sometimes gets to me and can make me feel stressed and anxious if I'm not performing well. I realise now that I used to turn to food to make me feel better if practice wasn't going well, or as a crutch if I lost a match. I'd often need something to settle me down; it could be food, drink, exercise – anything to take the edge off. In my mind, if I was eating extra food rather than taking drugs, I was doing well, and I'd pat myself on the back for taking the 'healthy' choice. I thought I wasn't doing harm to myself, but I was.

IT'S ALL ABOUT GAINING CONTROL over situations that could have been uncontrollable – and that's what this plan has given me. I won four tournaments, back-to-back, in the six months after starting this plan; I don't just put that down to ability – it's all about my frame of mind and the good foods that were feeding my brain.

I FEEL SO MUCH YOUNGER! Recently I did twelve weeks on the road and after eight weeks, 26 year olds were telling me that they were exhausted, burnt out and lacking focus, while I felt as fresh as a daisy! Obviously winning snooker matches was helping, but my mindset was on point and that was all thanks to my diet – the food I was eating was keeping me sharp.

IT'S NOT ABOUT FALLING DOWN – it's about getting up again, and I'm good at that.

MY KITCHEN TIPS

- Consistency is the key, so stick to your plan.

- Keep a food diary. If I eat too many biscuits, I make a note and put a sad face next to it, because that's how I feel afterwards!

- Rice is a staple food in my diet but it's a total pain to cook every day. I cook a big batch that will last me two to three days.

- At the start of each day I think, 'What's the thing that's going to take the most time to prepare?' and I make sure I do that first. Little changes like this will help you manage your time.

- Pre-mix your favourite spice blends in big batches to save time – you can then label and freeze them, either in big portions or in ice cube trays.

- Batch cook your main meals with extra portions and freeze some of them for another time.

- Write a weekly shopping list, planning your meals and snacks for the week ahead.

- Keep the shelf where you keep herb and spices well-stocked – it's so easy to give food a bit of a kick with some crushed chilli or other spices.

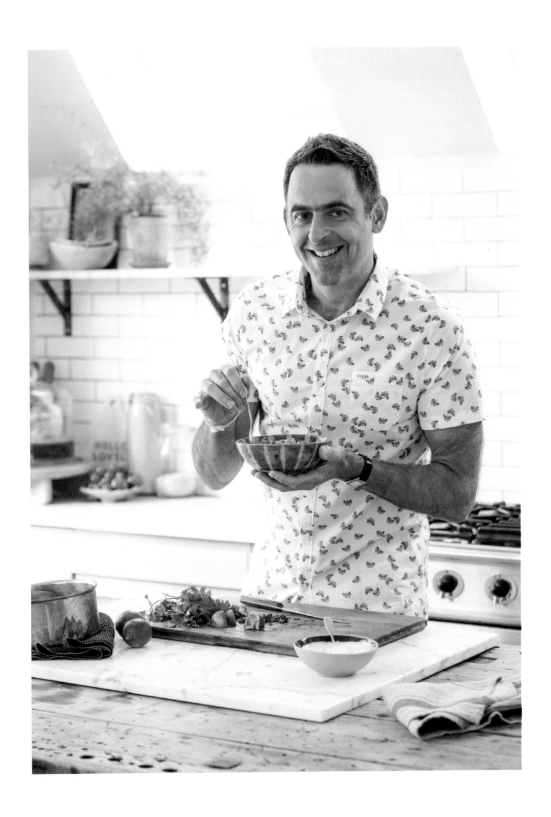

CONCLUSION

We live in a culture where everyone is stretched and stressed, but if we remember that the effort is ours to make, we can carve out the life we want. I don't want people to read this book and think, 'It's okay for him to preach – he probably has a chef, a driver and a personal trainer'. I don't actually have people to do things for me – I train myself, cook my own food and look after my kids. Being healthy and there for my kids is what matters most to me; everything else, snooker included, comes second.

No one will die if you don't answer your emails immediately – sometimes I just leave my phone in my car's glovebox and try to get away from the all-consuming noise, or I write a single email at the end of a day that rounds everything up. I have realised that I need peace of mind and focus in order to train and exist. To relax, I love to turn off my phone, cook and enjoy some quiet time.

I put my mind and my health first now – no one else is going to care about me more than I do, which is something I've learned the hard way. You need to care about yourself, it's just about finding the best people to help you do that. Don't get sucked into these faddy diets with their impossible promises; what you need is expert advice. I'm so grateful to Rhiannon for teaching me what I needed to know, and I hope I can help you now by passing on what I've learned.

RECIPES WITH RHIANNON

Remember, it's impossible to eat perfectly (whatever that means to you) all the time, but as soon as you've grasped the idea of nourishing your mind and body, soon enough, the tips and tricks Ronnie has learned with me will become second nature to you, helping you to become the healthiest version of yourself.

I really do believe that getting back to basics and keeping nutrition simple is the easiest way to maintain a healthy lifestyle. So, Ronnie and I want you to eat foods that help you to feel good and keep you energised, all while enjoying every morsel of food you eat.

The recipes I have created, inspired by Ronnie's travels and love for food from all around the world, don't make for a new diet, they're just full of nutrient-rich, energy-sustaining foods that'll keep you going all day long.

You'll find his favourite fry-ups, curries, pizzas and all sorts of foods you may think are typically unhealthy. Far from being disastrous for your body, these will quickly become your go-to meals, made with satisfying and fresh ingredients that won't break the bank. What's more, they're balanced with nutrition at their core, and with both meat and vegetarian options, they'll satisfy your body's every need without using numbers to guide you.

RECIPES

BREAKFAST

FRESH BREAKFAST BOWL

Don't be put off by its vivid green colour – this breakfast bowl tastes incredible and is full of power foods that will help you get through the day.

SERVES 1

1 banana
2 handfuls of spinach
½ ripe avocado
220ml milk of your choice
100g oats
6 ice cubes

Toppings:
80g fresh berries
20g dried coconut flakes
30g mixed nuts

1. Place all the ingredients in a blender and pulse until the mixture is smooth.

2. Serve topped with the fresh berries, coconut flakes and mixed nuts.

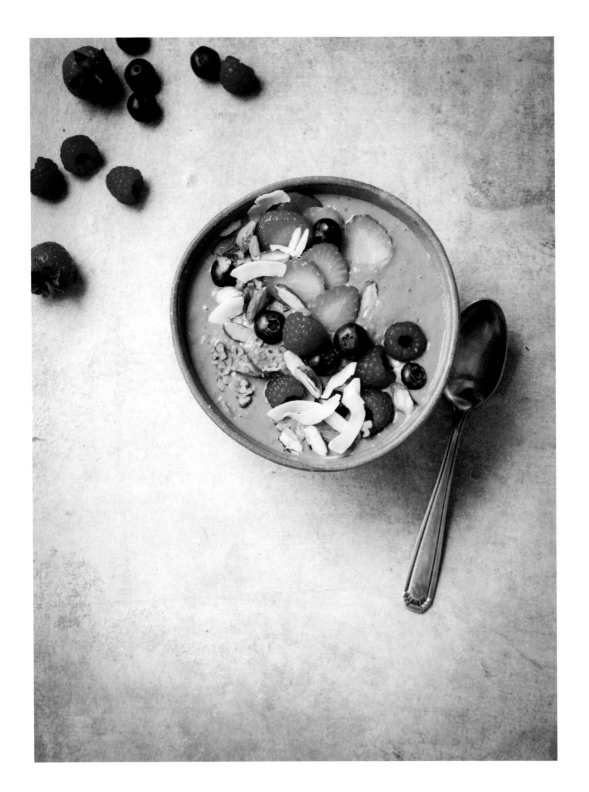

BANANA PORRIDGE

Bananas are a great source of energy and add a natural sweetness to your morning porridge. Walnuts contain more omega-3 fatty acids than any other nuts, making this porridge both tasty and nutritious.

SERVES 1

60g oats
½ tsp cinnamon
220ml milk of your choice
1 banana
30g walnuts, chopped

1. Heat the oats, cinnamon and milk in a saucepan over a low heat and stir until creamy.

2. Cut the banana in two. Mash one half of it and mix into the porridge. Cut the other half into thin slices and set aside.

3. Once the oats are cooked, pour into a bowl and top with the sliced banana and chopped walnuts.

BERRY PORRIDGE

You just can't go wrong with porridge — it's so simple and speedy to make. If you don't have fresh berries, frozen ones work nicely, too — just grab a handful from the freezer and either stir them into the porridge as it's cooking or scatter them on top at the end.

SERVES 1

60g oats
220ml almond milk
A scoop of protein powder
80g mixed fresh berries

1. Heat the oats, almond milk and protein powder in a saucepan over a low heat and stir until creamy.

2. Pour into a bowl and top with the mixed berries.

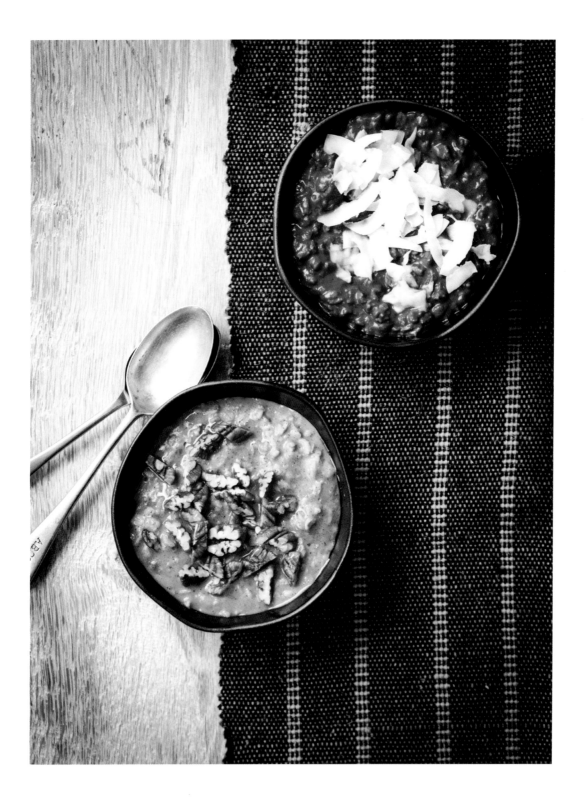

GINGERBREAD PORRIDGE

You can use any milk you like in this porridge — we especially like using oat milk.
If, like Ronnie and me, you like a bit of spice, this will be the breakfast for you!
It feels like a warming and sweet treat but doesn't contain any refined sugar.

SERVES 1

60g oats
2 tsp ground ginger
1 tsp cinnamon
220ml milk of your
choice
A handful of pecan
nuts, roughly chopped
(optional)
1 tsp honey (to serve)

1. Heat the oats, ground ginger, cinnamon and milk in a saucepan over a low heat and stir until creamy.

2. Pour into a bowl, top with the nuts and drizzle with honey.

CHOCOLATE PORRIDGE

Who doesn't love chocolate? This porridge is one of Ronnie's favourites — it's full
of cocoa but it's still healthy, with lots of fibre to keep you full until lunchtime.

SERVES 1

60g oats
2 tbsp cocoa powder
1 banana, mashed
220ml almond milk
A handful of dried
coconut flakes (optional)

1. Heat the oats, cocoa powder, mashed banana and milk in a saucepan over a low heat, and stir until creamy.

2. Pour into a bowl and top with the coconut flakes.

CHEESE PORRIDGE

Not everyone likes a sweet start to the morning, and this cheesy porridge is an amazing alternative. Ronnie says it tastes like dough balls with melted cheese!

SERVES 1

60g oats

220ml milk of your choice

1 tbsp lemon juice

30g Cheddar, grated

Salt and pepper

1. Heat the oats and milk in a saucepan over a low heat, and stir until creamy. Add the lemon juice and grated Cheddar and continue to stir, until the cheese melts.

2. Pour into a bowl and add salt and pepper to taste.

EGG MUFFINS

These muffins are a good source of protein and a great way to get some vegetables into your diet. They can be served warm from the oven or eaten cold on the go, making them really convenient on the days where you don't have much time.

SERVES 3

6 eggs
2 tbsp olive oil, plus extra for greasing
¼ onion, finely chopped
30g tomatoes, diced
¼ red pepper, finely chopped
6 button mushrooms, sliced
A handful of spinach, finely chopped

1. Preheat the oven to 180°C/Fan 160°C/Gas Mark 4.

2. Grease 6 muffin tin holes with olive oil. Beat the eggs and set aside.

3. Heat the olive oil in a saucepan over a medium heat. Add the onion, tomatoes, pepper, mushrooms and spinach.

4. Cook for 5–10 minutes until the vegetables become soft and take off the heat. Pour over the eggs and mix well.

5. Pour the mixture into the prepared muffin tin.

6. Bake in the oven for 20–25 minutes, until the eggs are set. Allow to cool for 10–15 minutes before serving.

BREAKFAST PANCAKES

Ronnie loves pancakes and wanted to create something that he could eat every morning without compromising his health. We devised this simple and nourishing recipe that will also provide some of your five a day.

SERVES 1

1 egg
1 banana, mashed
80g spelt flour
1 tsp cinnamon
100ml almond milk
80g blueberries
1 tbsp coconut oil
80g Greek yoghurt
1 tbsp honey

1. Combine the egg, banana, flour, cinnamon and almond milk in a bowl, and whisk until smooth. Stir half the blueberries into the mixture.

2. Place a frying pan over a medium heat and grease with coconut oil. Spoon the mixture onto the pan, making small pancakes.

3. Cook for 2–3 minutes on each side, or until golden.

4. Stack the pancakes on a plate and serve with the Greek yoghurt, the rest of the blueberries and a drizzle of honey.

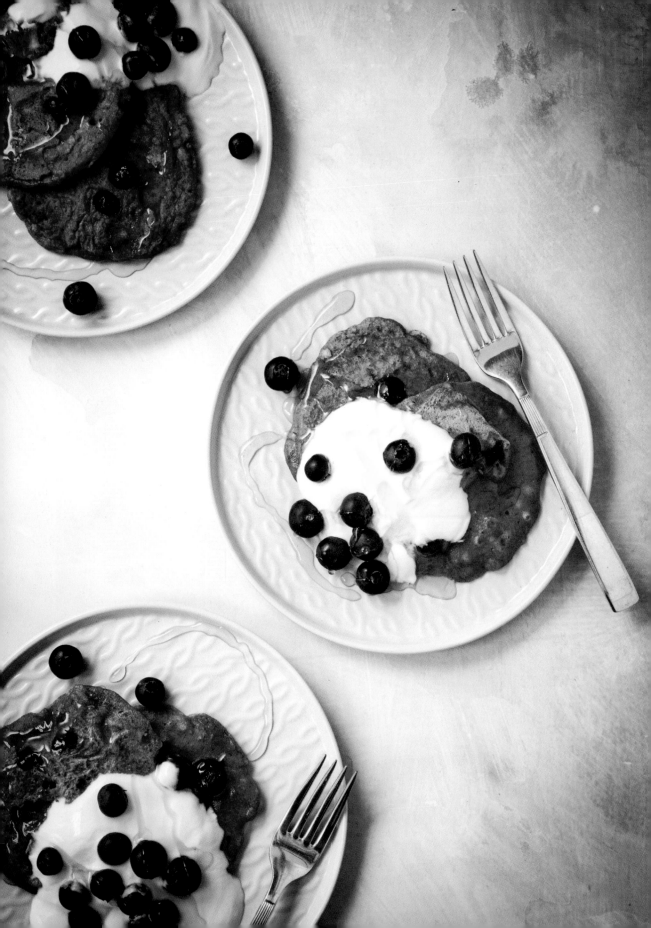

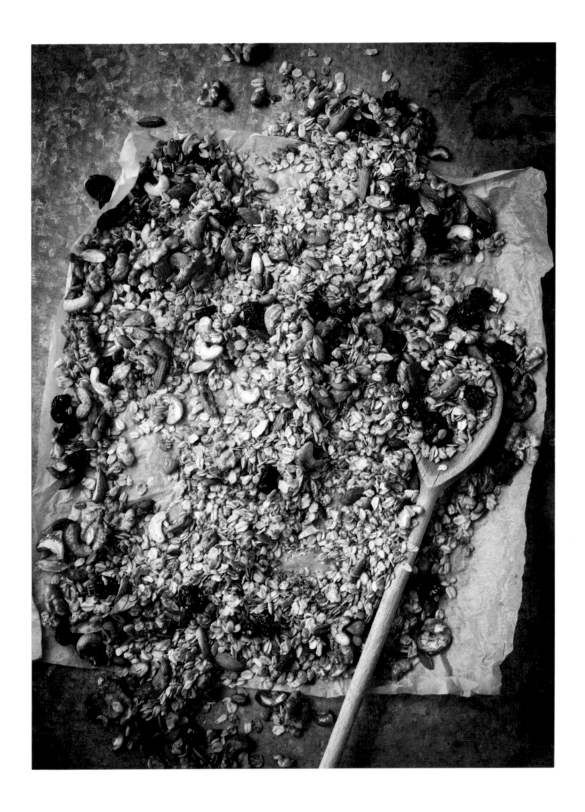

GRANOLA

Granola doesn't have to be full of sugar to taste great, and it will last for about a week in an airtight container. Serve it in a bowl with Greek yoghurt, some berries and topped with a drizzle of honey.

SERVES 2

160g oats
15g pumpkin seeds
30g almonds
30g cashews
30g walnuts
2 tbsp coconut oil, melted
3 tbsp honey
50g raisins

1. Preheat the oven to 180°C/Fan 160°C/Gas Mark 4.

2. Line a baking tray with baking paper. Combine all the ingredients, except the raisins, in a bowl. Use your hands to mix well, coating everything in the coconut oil and honey.

3. Spread the mixture on the prepared baking tray in a thin layer and bake in the oven for 20 minutes, stirring after 10 minutes to ensure that the ingredients toast evenly.

4. Allow to cool and mix in the raisins.

5. Serve with milk or yoghurt.

CHIA SEED RASPBERRY JAM ON TOAST

Chia seed jam has been a revelation for Ronnie – it contains far less refined sugar than shop-bought jam and is also far tastier. It's delicious on toast, muffins, yoghurt or in your porridge.

SERVES 4

200g raspberries
3 tbsp maple syrup
1 tsp lemon juice
3 tbsp chia seeds
2 slices of wholemeal toast

1. Set a saucepan over a medium heat and add the raspberries, maple syrup and lemon juice.

2. Bring the mixture to the boil, and continue to heat until it begins to break down and has a saucy consistency – this should take around 10 minutes.

3. Stir in the chia seeds and let the jam cook for another minute or so. Stir again, remove from the heat and leave it to thicken, which will take about 10 minutes.

4. Serve the jam hot or cold on wholemeal toast.

5. To store, place in a sterilised jam jar or other airtight container. It will keep in the fridge for up to two weeks.

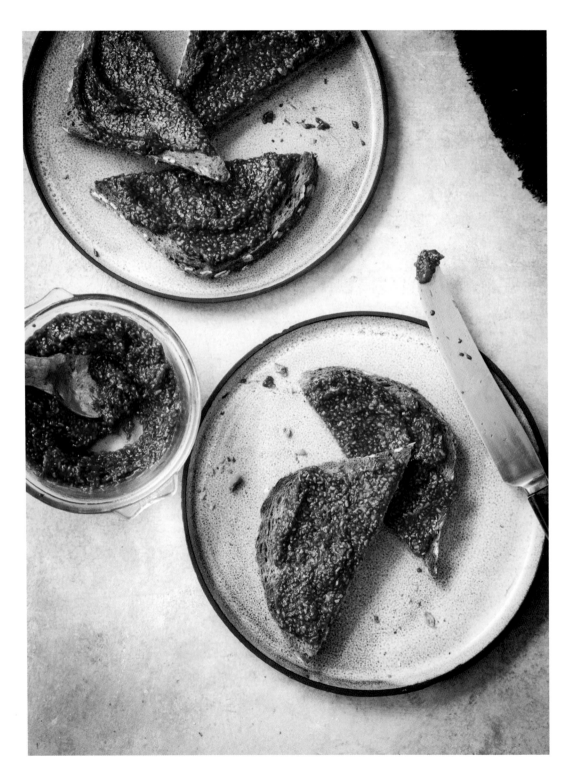

BREAKFAST OMELETTE

This omelette is one of the first things that I showed Ronnie how to make. It's a great way to get more vegetables in your diet and is now a firm favourite in his household. Don't be afraid to get creative and add any leftover vegetables that are lurking in the fridge!

SERVES 1

3 eggs
Salt and pepper
1 tbsp olive oil
3 small mushrooms, sliced
20g mozzarella or Cheddar cheese, grated
A handful of spinach

1. Whisk the eggs with the salt and pepper and set aside. Set a frying pan over a medium heat and grease with olive oil.

2. Pour the beaten eggs into the pan and cook for a minute or so, until the edges start to set. Add the sliced mushrooms, grated cheese and spinach.

3. Cook for a couple of minutes, until the centre begins to set. Fold the omelette in half and leave on the heat for another minute or so, and then slide it onto a plate.

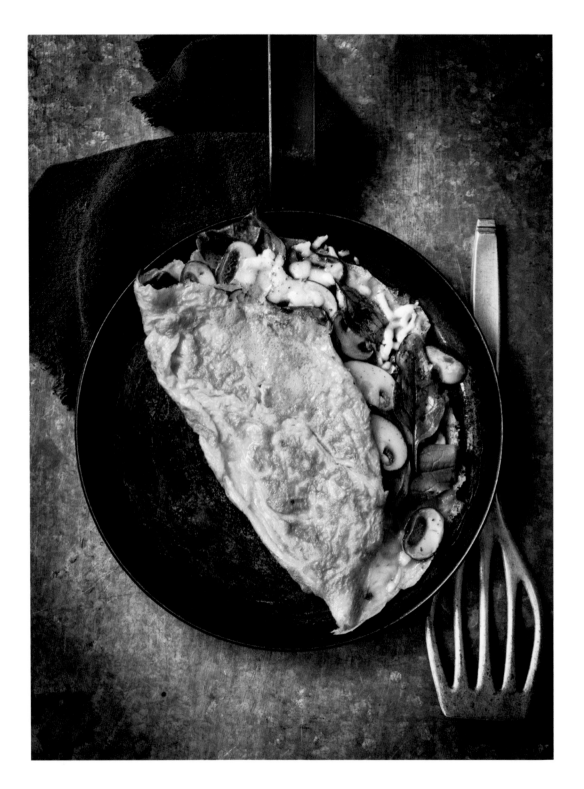

FRENCH TOAST

This is the ultimate weekend breakfast and Ronnie always looks forward to it the morning after a match. It contains fibre, fruit and healthy fat, and there's plenty of protein in the nut butter and eggs. It may seem indulgent, but it contains everything he needs before he goes on a late-morning run.

SERVES 2

4 slices of wholemeal bread
½ banana, thinly sliced
2 tbsp peanut butter
60ml almond milk
2 eggs
½ tsp vanilla essence
½ tsp cinnamon
1 tbsp coconut oil
2 tbsp maple syrup
80g fresh berries

1. First, make two peanut butter and banana sandwiches.

2. Then, whisk together the almond milk, eggs, vanilla extract and cinnamon. Pour the mixture into a container large enough to fit the sandwiches and soak each one on both sides for about 10 seconds.

3. Preheat a frying pan over a medium-high heat and grease with the coconut oil, to prevent the sandwiches from sticking. Cook each one for 3–4 minutes on each side, or until golden.

4. Cut each sandwich in half, drizzle with maple syrup and finish with the fresh berries.

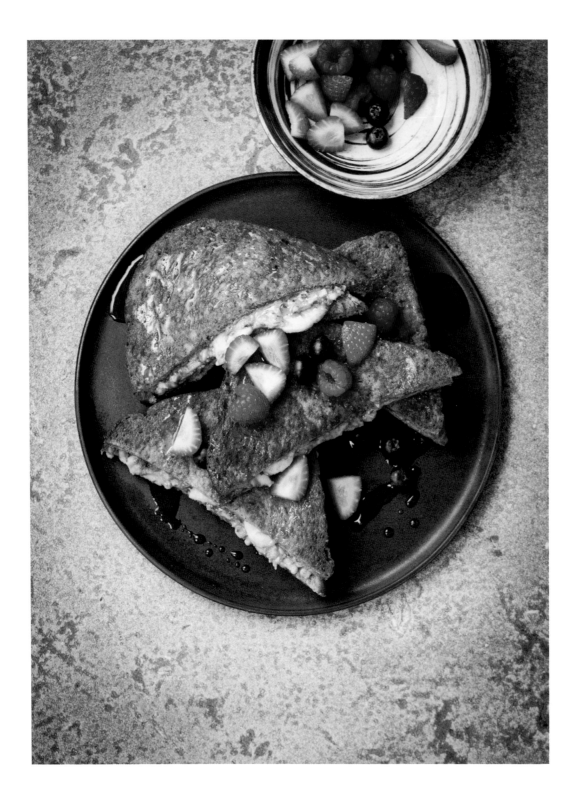

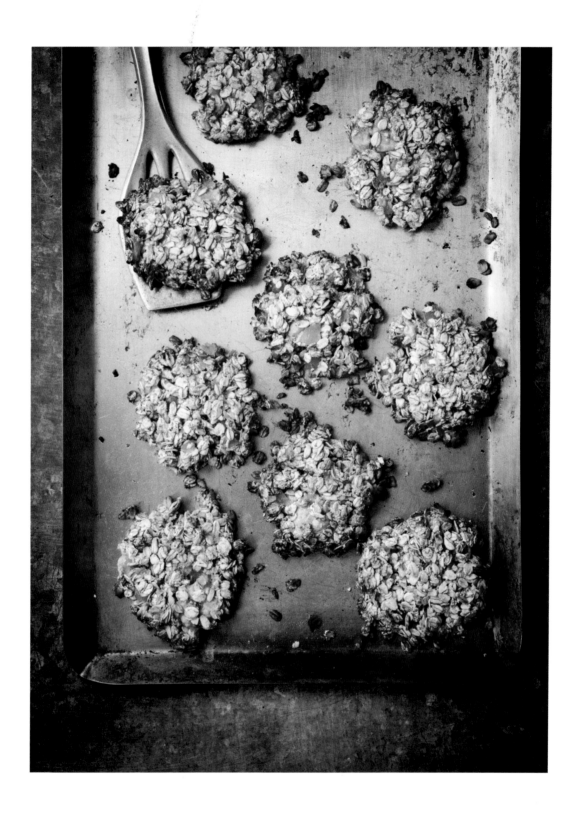

BANANA AND CINNAMON BREAKFAST COOKIES

If you're too busy to make breakfast, we have the answer! Make a batch of these at the weekend and keep them in an airtight container – they will ensure you can eat a healthy breakfast on the go!

SERVES 4

220g oats
2 ripe bananas, mashed
120g unsweetened
apple sauce
1 tsp cinnamon
1 tsp vanilla extract

1. Preheat the oven to 200°C/Fan 180°C/Gas Mark 6.

2. Line a baking tray with baking paper. Mix all the ingredients in a bowl, until combined.

3. Divide the mixture into around 12 cookie shapes on the prepared baking tray, spaced well apart.

4. Bake for 20–25 minutes in the oven, until golden.

5. Allow to cool for 5–10 minutes before eating.

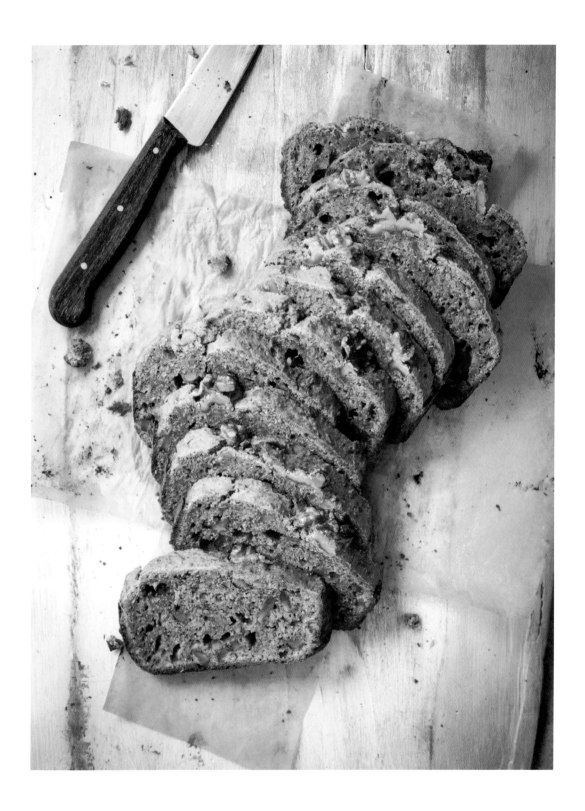

BANANA BREAD

The smell of freshly baked banana bread is second-to-none, and this recipe is so easy to make. You can enjoy it either on its own or topped with a dollop of yoghurt and peanut butter. If you have any overripe bananas in your fruit bowl, this is the perfect way to use them up.

SERVES 6

240g wholemeal flour
1 tsp baking powder
2 eggs
2 ripe bananas, mashed
50g honey
4 tbsp coconut oil, melted
1 tsp vanilla extract
50g Greek yoghurt
50g walnuts, chopped

1. Preheat the oven to 200°C/180°C fan/Gas Mark 6.

2. Line a 1-litre bread tin with baking paper, or alternatively grease with coconut oil.

3. Mix the flour and baking powder in a bowl. In a separate bowl, whisk together the eggs, mashed banana, honey, melted coconut oil, vanilla extract and yoghurt until the mixture is smooth.

4. Stir the dry mixture into the wet mixture and add the chopped walnuts.

5. Pour the mixture into the loaf tin and bake in the oven for 45–50 minutes, until it is firm to the touch. If a knife inserted into the centre comes out clean, it's ready.

6. Allow to cool for 10–15 minutes and serve hot or cold.

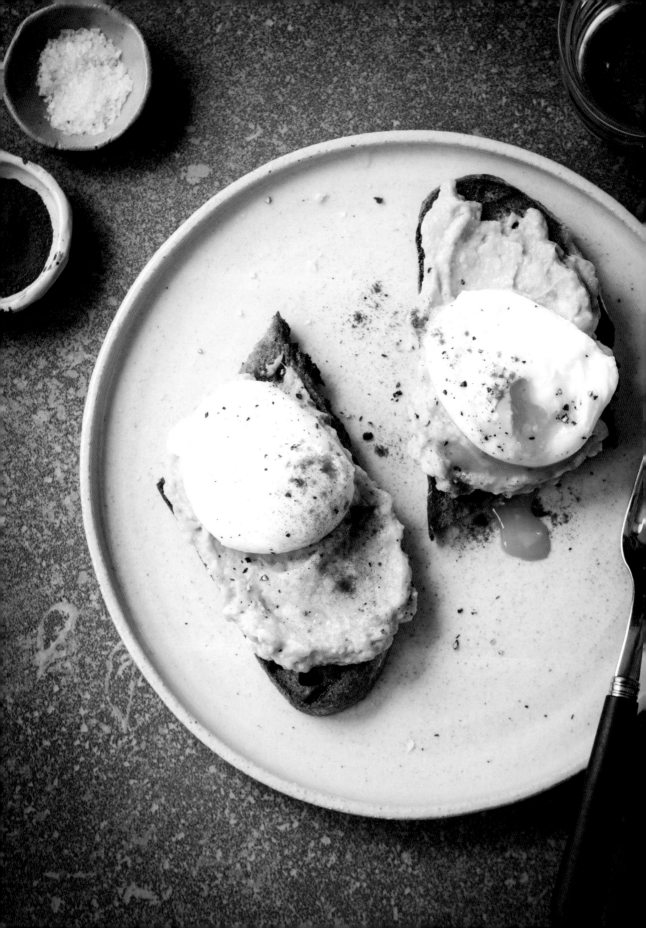

POACHED EGGS ON RYE BREAD WITH AVOCADO

This is a simple and tasty breakfast or brunch that will please everyone. It's great with any bread but we've used rye bread here – because it's sturdy, your eggs and avocado will sit nicely on the toast.

SERVES 1

2 slices of rye bread
2 eggs
½ avocado
½ tsp smoked paprika
Salt

1. Bring a small saucepan of water to the boil. Meanwhile, toast the rye bread for 3–4 minutes.

2. With the water on a light boil, break the eggs into a ramekin and gently pour each one into the water.

3. Time the eggs for 3 ½–4 minutes.

4. Mash the avocado onto the toast.

5. Scoop the eggs out of the water – they should still feel soft in the middle, though the whites should be solid – and place on top of the avocado.

6. Sprinkle with smoked paprika and a pinch of salt.

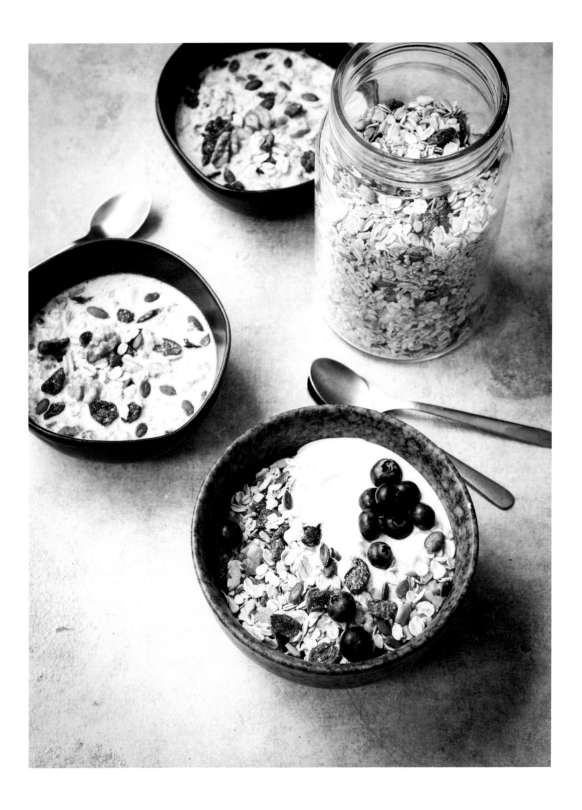

CINNAMON MUESLI

This muesli is wonderful on its own or sprinkled on top of fruit and yoghurt.

SERVES 6

400g oats
100g mixed seeds
150g walnuts, chopped
100g dried cranberries
2 tsp cinnamon

1. Combine all the ingredients in a jar and shake well.

2. Serve with either milk or natural yoghurt.

FLATBREAD AND HUMMUS

We wanted to think outside the box and include a breakfast idea that was a bit different! This hummus is simple and tasty and goes fantastically with homemade flatbreads, making a great snack or a tasty addition to a main meal.

SERVES 4

For the flatbread:
250g wholemeal self-raising flour
1 tsp baking powder
½ tsp sea salt
250g natural yoghurt

For the hummus:
400g chickpeas
3 tbsp olive oil
3 tbsp tahini
1 tbsp lemon juice
½ tsp sea salt
½ tsp ground black pepper

1. Mix together the flour, baking powder and salt, and stir in the yoghurt. Mix with your hands or a spoon, until it forms a dough-like mixture.

2. Place the dough on a floured surface and knead for 2–3 minutes. Separate it into 6 pieces and roll them into circles.

3. Heat a large frying pan and add one flatbread at a time, cooking for 2 minutes on each side, before removing from the pan and allowing to cool.

4. Drain and rinse the chickpeas. For a smoother hummus, remove the skins from the chickpeas.

5. Combine the chickpeas, olive oil, tahini, lemon juice, salt and pepper in a blender. Blend for 1–2 minutes until the mixture is completely smooth.

6. Transfer to a bowl and serve with the flatbreads.

BREAKFAST PITTA SANDWICH

This savoury breakfast is a really handy option. You can make it the night before and keep it in the fridge, so it's ready to grab in the morning.

SERVES 1

1 wholemeal pitta bread
2 eggs
1 tbsp olive oil
30g feta, crumbled
4 cherry tomatoes, chopped
1 handful of spinach leaves

1. Toast the pitta bread and then slice it along the long side, so you can fill it.

2. Beat the eggs in a cup. Heat a small saucepan over a medium heat, greasing with olive oil.

3. Pour the eggs into the pan and scramble them. Once they begin to cook, add the feta, tomatoes and spinach leaves.

4. Continue to stir the mixture until cooked and then use it to fill the pitta bread pocket.

PEANUT BUTTER SMOOTHIE

A smoothie can be the quickest way to get some goodness before you leave the house in the morning. This peanut butter version tastes a bit like ice cream – it's completely delicious!

SERVES 1

1 banana
100ml milk of
your choice
60g Greek yoghurt
40g oats
2 tbsp peanut butter,
smooth or crunchy
½ tsp cinnamon
5 ice cubes

1. Add all the ingredients to a blender and blend until smooth and creamy. Pour into a glass.

GREEN SMOOTHIE

Don't be put off by the vegetables that are in this smoothie – the banana and berries overpower the taste of the kale and spinach, making it a wonderful way of incorporating more veg into your diet without you even noticing!

SERVES 1

1 banana
A handful of spinach
A handful of kale
40g blueberries
40g oats
100ml coconut water
5 ice cubes

1. Add all the ingredients to a blender and blend until smooth. Pour into a glass.

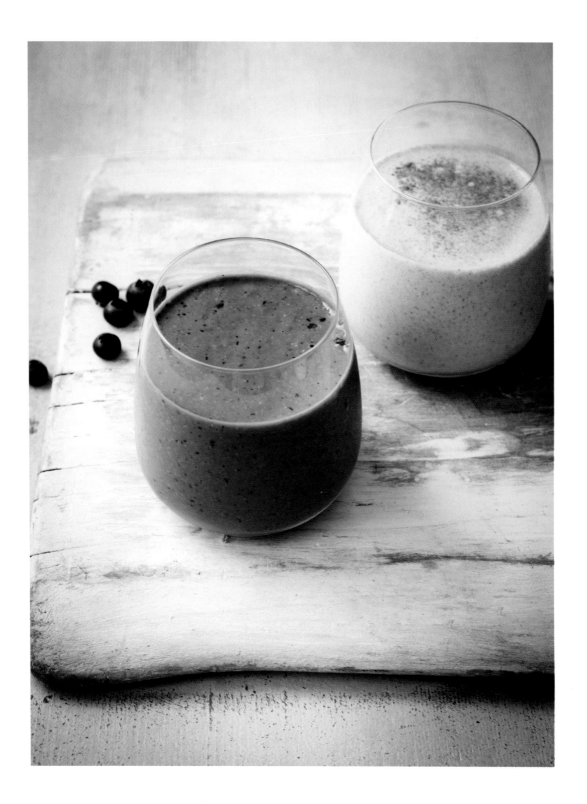

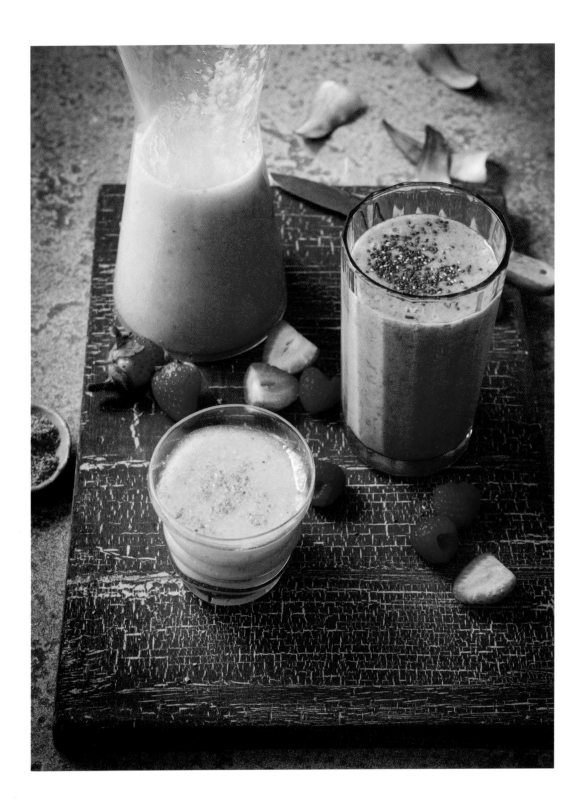

TROPICAL SMOOTHIE

If you want to vary your morning routine, give this smoothie a try. Ronnie is a big fan of trying different flavours and often makes this fruity concoction.

SERVES 1

1 orange, peeled
1 banana, peeled
200ml coconut water
60g mango, cut into chunks
60g pineapple, cut into chunks
1 tbsp chia seeds or ground flaxseed
5 ice cubes

1. Add all the ingredients to a blender and blend until smooth. Pour into a glass.

BERRY SMOOTHIE

This smoothie is a delicious and nourishing way to enjoy your breakfast. Frozen berries are more cost-effective than fresh ones and retain all the nutritional benefits.

SERVES 1

1 banana
200ml almond milk
80g mixed berries
1 tsp chia seeds or ground flaxseed
5 ice cubes

1. Add all the ingredients to a blender and blend until smooth. Pour into a glass.

STRAWBERRY MANGO SMOOTHIE

A delicious fruity start to the day, this smoothie is rich in Vitamin C and fibre, which helps to keep you fit and healthy.

SERVES 1

1 banana
40g oats
40g mango, cut into chunks
40g strawberries
1 tbsp honey
5 ice cubes

1. Add all the ingredients to a blender and blend until smooth. Pour into a glass.

CLASSIC OVERNIGHT OATS

Overnight oats are a great option for hurried mornings. Just pop them in the fridge the night before you want them for breakfast and you can eat them on the way to work.

SERVES 1

50g Greek yoghurt
40g oats
150ml milk of your choice
1 tbsp chia seeds
1 tbsp honey

1. Mix the ingredients in a bowl until combined and spoon into an airtight jar.

2. Leave in the fridge overnight (or for at least 4 hours) before eating.

CINNAMON SPICE OVERNIGHT OATS

If you're in need of a delicious, cooling treat to start your day, these cinnamon spice overnight oats will transform your morning routine. Prepare them the night before and top with extra fruit for extra sweetness.

SERVES 1

50g Greek yoghurt
40g oats
150ml milk of your choice
1 tbsp chia seeds
1 tbsp honey or maple syrup
1 tsp cinnamon
½ tsp nutmeg
½ tsp ground ginger

1. Mix all the ingredients in a bowl until combined and spoon into an airtight jar.

2. Leave in the fridge overnight (or for at least 4 hours) before eating.

CHOCOLATE AND COCONUT OVERNIGHT OATS

The flavours of chocolate and coconut go really nicely together. Try throwing in some additional berries if you have any in the fridge!

SERVES 1

50g Greek yoghurt
40g oats
150ml coconut milk
1 tbsp chia seeds
1 tbsp honey or maple syrup
2 tbsp cocoa powder
2 tbsp dried coconut flakes

1. Mix all the ingredients in a bowl until combined and spoon into an airtight jar.

2. Leave in the fridge overnight (or for at least 4 hours) before eating.

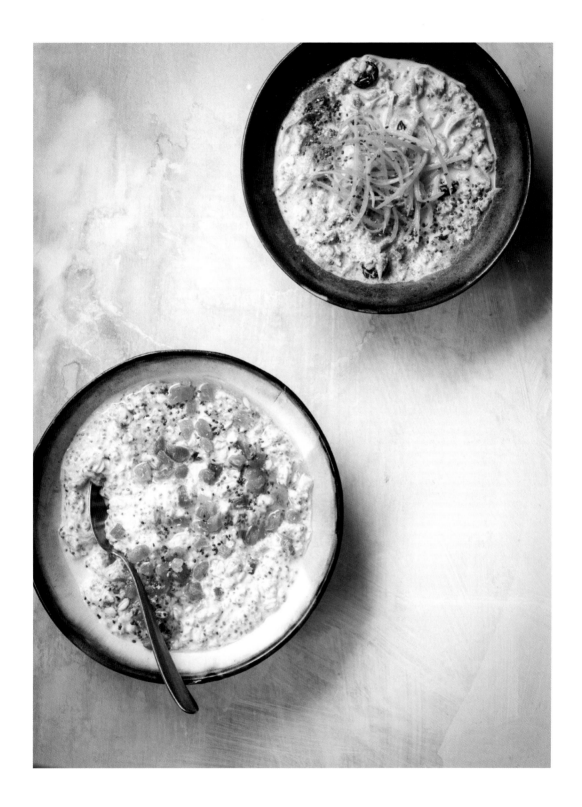

APRICOT OVERNIGHT OATS

Grab-and-go breakfasts can be essential when you have a hectic schedule. Apricots are an excellent source of Vitamin A and a good source of Vitamin C to help keep you healthy.

SERVES 1

50g Greek yoghurt

40g oats

150ml milk of your choice

1 tbsp chia seeds

1 tbsp honey or maple syrup

40g dried apricots, chopped

1. Mix all the ingredients in a bowl until combined and spoon into an airtight jar.

2. Leave in the fridge overnight (or for at least 4 hours) before eating.

CARROT CAKE OVERNIGHT OATS

These speedy and delicious oats really do taste like carrot cake – who says breakfast needs to be boring?

SERVES 1

50g Greek yoghurt

40g oats

150ml milk of your choice

1 tbsp chia seeds

1 tbsp honey or maple syrup

1 carrot, grated

30g raisins

½ tsp cinnamon

½ tsp vanilla extract

1. Mix all the ingredients in a bowl until combined and spoon into an airtight jar.

2. Leave in the fridge overnight (or for at least 4 hours) before eating.

LUNCH

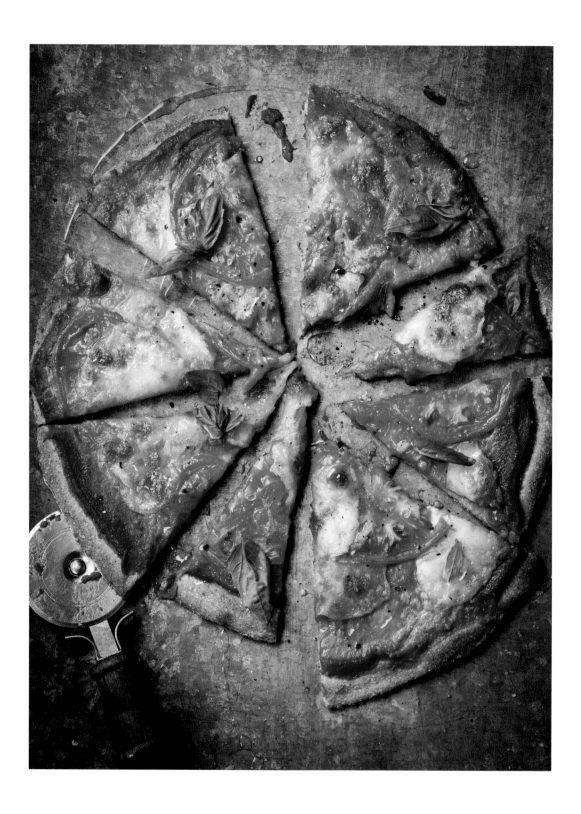

RONNIE AND RHIANNON'S HOMEMADE PIZZA

Pizza can be a balanced and healthy meal, if you use the right toppings and cook them from scratch. And making your own bases doesn't have to be complicated — you can get the whole family involved, or maybe even listen to music while you cook!

SERVES 2

For the pizza dough:

250g wholemeal self-raising flour

1 tsp baking powder

½ tsp sea salt

250g natural yoghurt

For the pizza topping:

150ml passata

2 tbsp tomato paste

2 large tomatoes, sliced

A handful of basil, chopped

125g mozzarella, sliced

1. Preheat the oven to 200°C/Fan 180°C/Gas Mark 6.

2. Line a baking try with baking paper.

3. Mix together the flour, baking powder and salt, and then stir in the yoghurt.

4. Mix either with your hands or a spoon until you start to achieve a dough-like mixture.

5. Knead the dough on a floured surface for 4–5 minutes. Use a floured rolling pin to roll the dough into 2 large circles.

6. Mix the passata with the tomato paste, spread the mixture across each pizza base and add your toppings.

7. Bake in the oven for 20–25 minutes, until the base is golden.

8. Remove from the oven, cut into slices and serve.

RAINBOW CHILLI STIR FRY

Having spent a lot of time playing snooker in China, Chinese food is one of Ronnie's favourite cuisines. He loves spice, but feel free to use as much or as little chilli as you like in this stir fry!

SERVES 2

A small bunch of fresh coriander

2 garlic cloves

1 fresh red chilli

200g chicken (or tofu for vegan option)

1 tbsp olive oil

50g cashew nuts

2 carrots, peeled and cut into julienne strips

80g broccoli, chopped

200g wholewheat noodles, cooked

2 tbsp soy sauce

A pinch of freshly ground black pepper

1 tbsp sesame seeds (optional)

1. Chop the coriander leaves finely. Peel and finely slice the garlic. Deseed and finely slice the chilli. Cut the chicken into strips (or, if using tofu, cut into small squares).

2. Heat a large frying pan over a medium-high heat, greasing with the olive oil. Add the cashew nuts, fry until lightly toasted and place on a plate.

3. Add the chicken (or tofu) to the pan and cook for 2–3 minutes. Add the garlic, carrots, broccoli and the cooked noodles. Add the soy sauce and stir until the chicken is completely cooked.

4. Remove from the heat and add to 2 bowls. Add the toasted nuts to each and finish off with coriander, chilli, black pepper and sesame seeds.

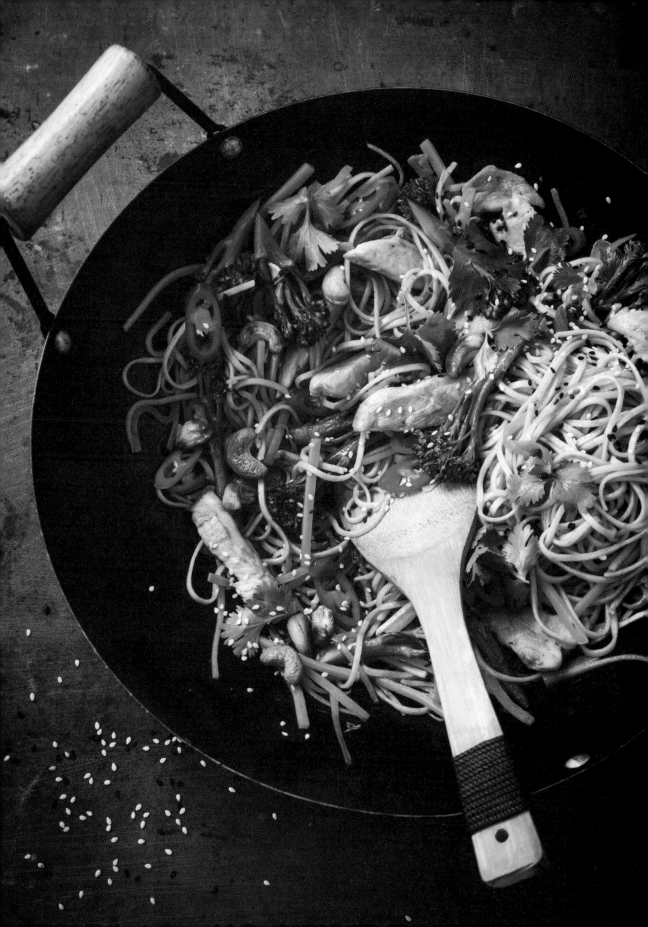

BLACK BEAN BURRITOS

We all lead busy lives and sometimes we get stuck in a rut, so I gave Ronnie some recipes for quick and simple burritos that he can take to snooker practice. These black bean ones taste amazing and are really quick to prepare.

SERVES 2

1 tbsp olive oil

½ garlic clove, crushed

200g black beans, drained

100g red kidney beans, drained

100ml water

½ tsp chipotle chilli powder

80g chopped plum tomatoes

2 tbsp red onion, thinly sliced

2 large wholemeal wraps

50g Cheddar, grated

2 tbsp soured cream

2 tbsp tomato salsa

40g romaine lettuce, shredded

1 tbsp coriander, roughly chopped

1. Heat the oil in a large pan over a medium heat. Add the garlic, black beans and kidney beans to the pan, add water and bring to boil. Stir in the chipotle chilli powder, add the tomatoes and onion, and simmer on a low heat for 10 minutes.

2. Heat the tortilla wraps in the microwave for 30 seconds and lay them on a plate.

3. Divide the bean mixture between the wraps and top each one with grated cheddar, soured cream, salsa and the shredded lettuce, before folding into a wrap.

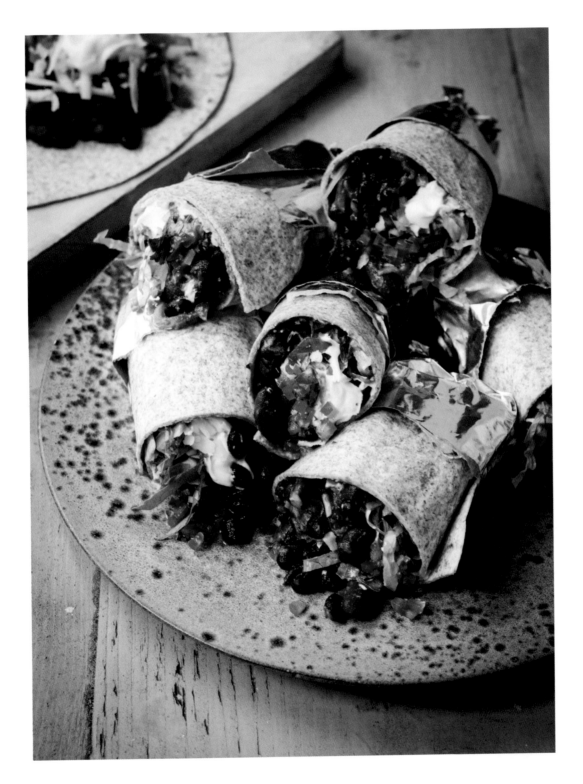

JACKET SWEET POTATO AND HOMEMADE BEANS

Ronnie loves a comforting meal and this classic 'spud and beans' recipe is one of his favourites.

SERVES 2

2 medium-sized sweet potatoes

1 tbsp olive oil

1 carrot, diced

200g haricot beans, drained

1 large tomato, chopped

1 tsp paprika

50ml water

1 tsp Worcestershire sauce

1. Preheat the oven to 200°C/Fan 180°C/Gas Mark 6.

2. Wash and dry the potatoes, before piercing each one several times with a fork. Bake in the oven for 1 hour, until they feel soft.

3. While the potatoes are cooking, heat the oil in a saucepan set over a medium heat and add the carrots. Cook for 5–10 minutes until soft.

4. Add the beans, tomato and paprika, and cook for a further 5 minutes until the tomatoes have softened. Stir in the water and Worcestershire sauce, and cook for another 5 minutes, stirring occasionally.

5. Turn the heat off and cover to keep warm. When the sweet potatoes are ready, split them open and dish the beans out evenly across each one.

BAKED FISH WITH HERBS

Simple, healthy and ready in less than five minutes, this is an excellent dish to cook when you're short of time.

SERVES 2

2 cod fillets (skin on)
1 tsp dried rosemary
1 tsp thyme leaves
A pinch of sea salt
½ tsp crushed black peppercorns
1 tbsp olive oil
1 lemon, thinly sliced

1. Preheat the oven to 200°C/Fan 180°C/Gas Mark 6.

2. Line a baking tray with foil or parchment paper and place the cod fillets on it, skin side down.

3. In a bowl, mix together the rosemary, thyme, sea salt and crushed black peppercorns, then spread the mixture across each fillet of fish. Drizzle with the olive oil, scatter the lemon slices across the top of each fish and fold the sides of the parchment paper over, creating a parcel for the fish.

4. Bake in the oven for 15 minutes or until the fish is cooked through.

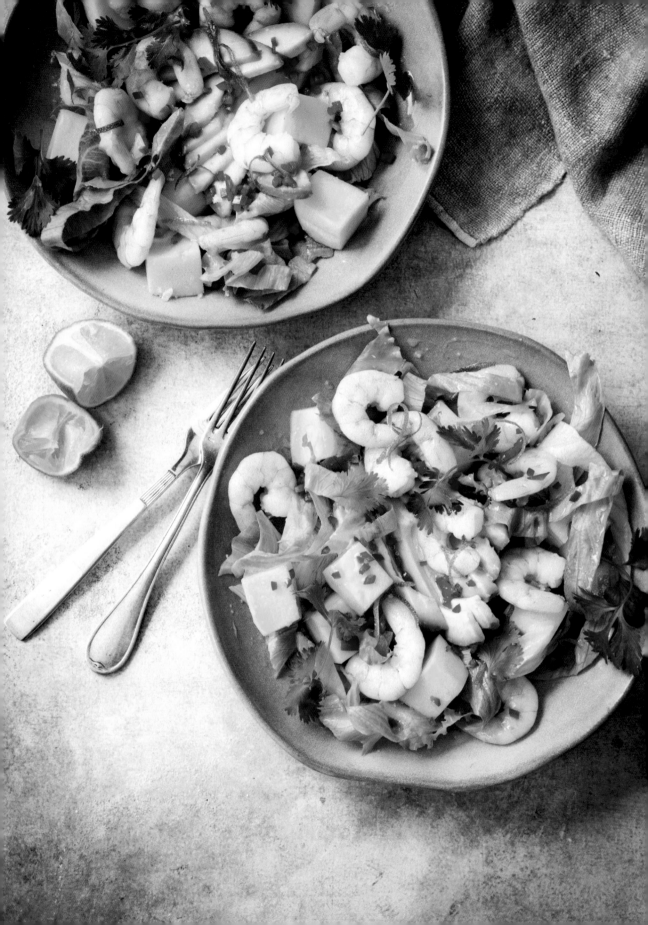

MANGO, PRAWN AND AVOCADO SALAD

This refreshing salad is wonderful by itself or as part of a bigger meal; it requires very little fuss, but packs in a lot of flavour.

SERVES 2

200g cooked tiger prawns

1 mango, chopped into cubes

1 avocado, sliced

1 lime

½ red chilli, deseeded and finely chopped

1 tbsp honey

1 tbsp avocado oil

½ iceberg lettuce, shredded

1. Place the prawns in a bowl with the chopped mango and avocado.

2. Add the zest and juice of half the lime to a bowl.

3. Mix with chilli, honey and oil. Cut the other half of the lime into wedges. Drizzle the dressing over the prawns, avocado and mango.

4. Serve on a bed of iceberg lettuce with a wedge of lime.

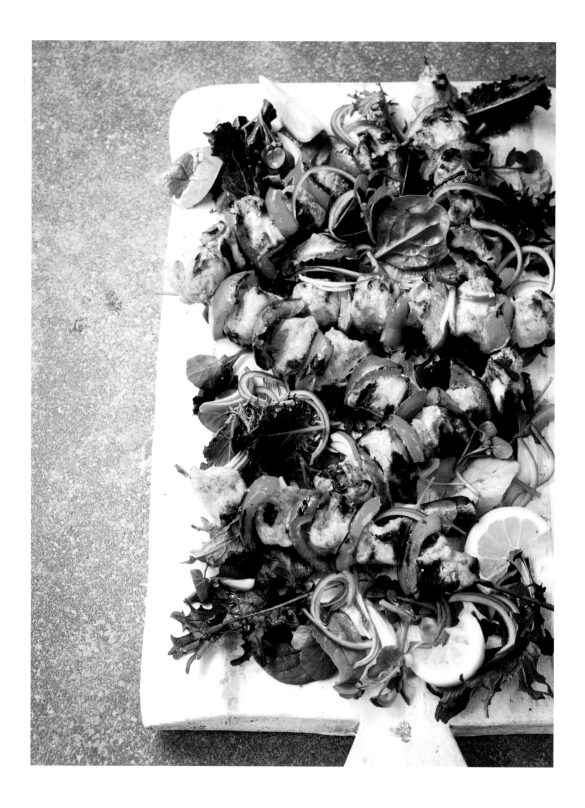

CHICKEN KEBABS

There's nothing more satisfying than a juicy kebab that's bursting with flavour. These are Ronnie's favourites and can be eaten hot or cold.

SERVES 4

12 wooden skewers

2 garlic cloves
140g natural yoghurt
60ml passata
2 tbsp olive oil
½ tsp ground ginger
½ tsp paprika
½ tsp ground turmeric
1 tsp garam masala
4 skinless chicken breasts
½ red pepper
½ green pepper

1. Place the wooden skewers in cold water to soak, which will stop them from burning.

2. Peel the garlic and grate into a mixing bowl. Add the yoghurt, passata, 1 tablespoon of the olive oil, the ground ginger, paprika, turmeric and garam masala and mix well.

3. Cut the chicken breasts into bite-sized chunks and add to the bowl. Toss the chicken to marinate and leave in the fridge for 2 hours. In the meantime, chop the peppers into bite-sized chunks.

4. Remove the skewers from the cold water and dry them.

5. Once the chicken is marinated, divide across the skewers, threading a piece of pepper for every piece of chicken (not too close together).

6. Place on a baking tray and cook under the grill for 10–15 minutes, turning every 2–3 minutes.

7. Serve with a green salad and pickled red onions.

CHICKEN SALAD SANDWICH WITH GREEK YOGHURT

This recipe takes a classic sandwich but adds more of the good stuff — the filling!
I know a sandwich can often lack protein and vegetables, so we developed a few twists.

SERVES 1

1 cooked chicken fillet, shredded

30g dried cranberries

½ apple, finely chopped

50g Greek yoghurt

2 large lettuce leaves

2 slices of wholemeal bread

1. Place the chicken, cranberries, apple and Greek yoghurt in a bowl and mix together.

2. Place the mixture on a slice of bread and top with the lettuce leaves.

3. Top with the second piece of bread and cut in half.

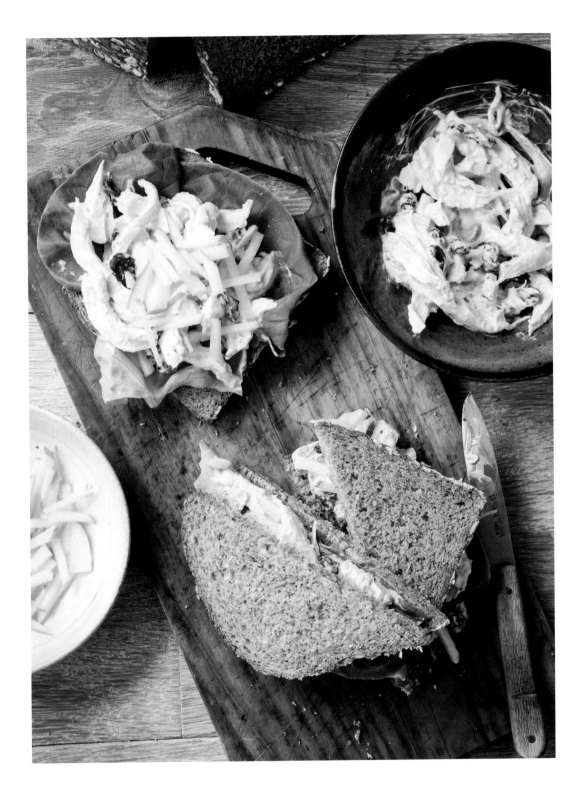

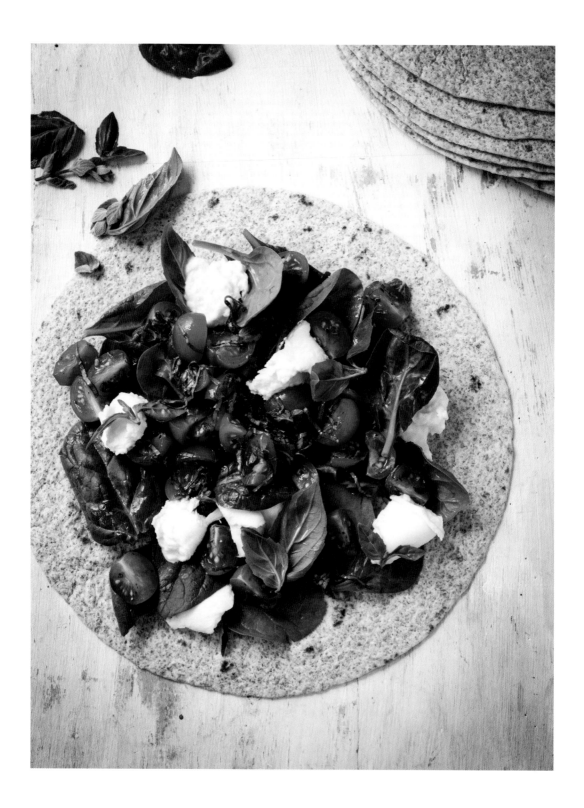

TOMATO AND MOZZARELLA PIZZA WRAPS

What could be better than pizza? How about a tasty wrap that's like a pizza but you can take it anywhere.

SERVES 2

12 cherry tomatoes, quartered

2 tbsp fresh basil, chopped

1 tbsp fresh oregano

80g spinach

50g mozzarella, sliced

2 wholemeal wraps

1. Combine the tomatoes, basil, oregano and spinach in a bowl.

2. Place the wraps flat on a plate and add the tomato. Mix evenly across each one.

3. Divide the mozzarella between the wraps and fold them up.

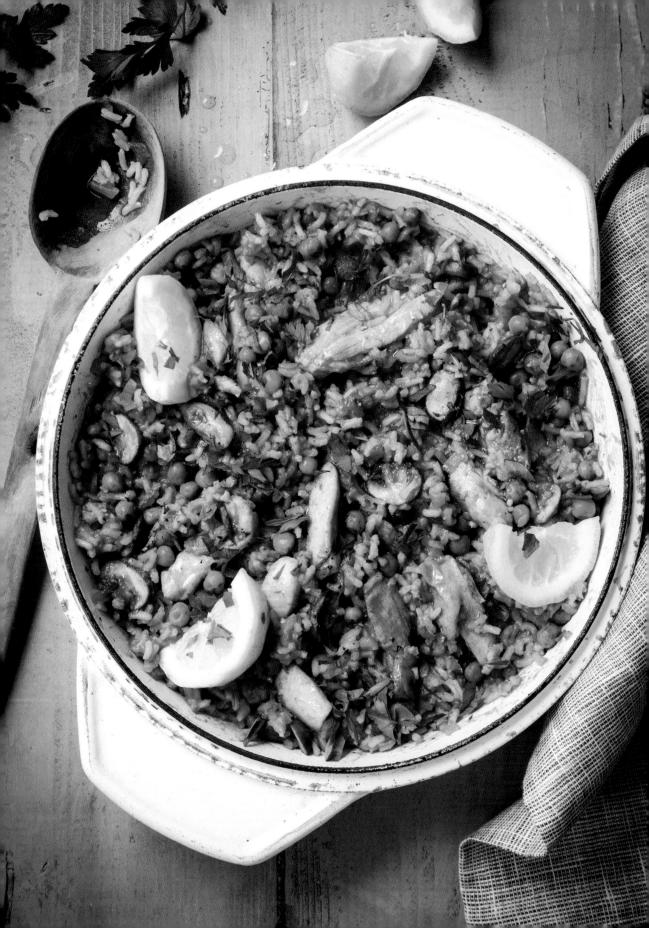

RONNIE'S PAELLA

Ronnie has loved paella ever since his best mate taught him to cook it and this recipe is a firm favourite in his household. Feel free to add any vegetables you like.

SERVES 2

1 tbsp olive oil

½ onion, chopped

14 button mushrooms, sliced

200g skinless chicken thigh fillets, cut into strips

1 garlic clove, crushed

1 tsp paprika

½ tsp turmeric

200g wholegrain rice

200g tinned chopped tomatoes

1 tbsp tomato puree

500ml chicken stock

80g frozen peas

A pinch of sea salt

1 tsp ground black pepper

Lemon wedges

1. Heat the olive oil in a large frying pan set over a medium heat. Add the onion and mushrooms and fry for 3 minutes. Add the chicken and fry for another 2–3 minutes. Add a little water if needed.

2. Add the garlic, paprika and turmeric and cook for another 2 minutes.

3. Stir in the rice until it is covered in the spices, then stir in the chopped tomatoes, tomato puree and chicken stock. Season and bring to the boil.

4. Cover the pan with a lid and continue to cook on a medium heat for 30 minutes. Add the frozen peas and cook for a further 5 minutes. Remove the pan from the heat and allow to stand for 5–10 minutes.

5. Divide the dish into two servings and garnish with the lemon wedges.

MISO AUBERGINE

I've been introducing Ronnie to different fermented foods and this miso aubergine recipe is our favourite vegetarian dish to make – it's very simple and tastes incredible. The miso is naturally sweet and adds a gorgeous texture to the aubergine.

SERVES 2

2 small aubergines,
halved lengthways
2 tbsp olive oil
50g brown miso
100g couscous
1 red chilli, thinly sliced
50g spinach
Salt and pepper

1. Preheat the oven to 200°C/Fan 180°C/Gas Mark 6.

2. Make criss-cross patterns across the inside of the sliced aubergines, brush the surface with olive oil and place on a baking tray.

3. Mix the brown miso with 20ml of water to create a thick paste. Spread across the aubergines, cover with foil and roast for 20–25 minutes in the oven. Remove the foil and roast for a further 10–15 minutes.

4. In the meantime, boil 200ml water in a saucepan, adding a pinch of salt.

5. In a separate pan, heat 1 tablespoon of olive oil and fry the couscous for 2 minutes. Then add it to the boiling water and cook for 10 minutes. Drain well and place on top of the aubergines.

6. Season and serve with the sliced chilli and spinach.

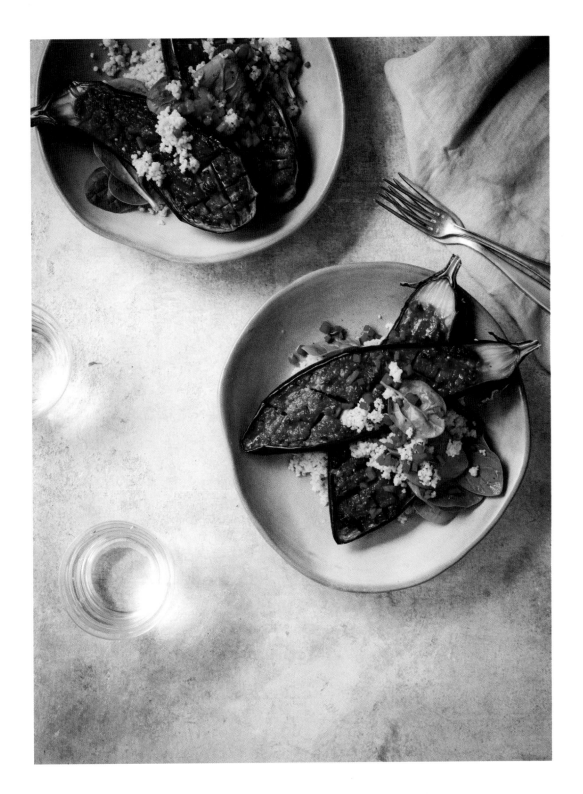

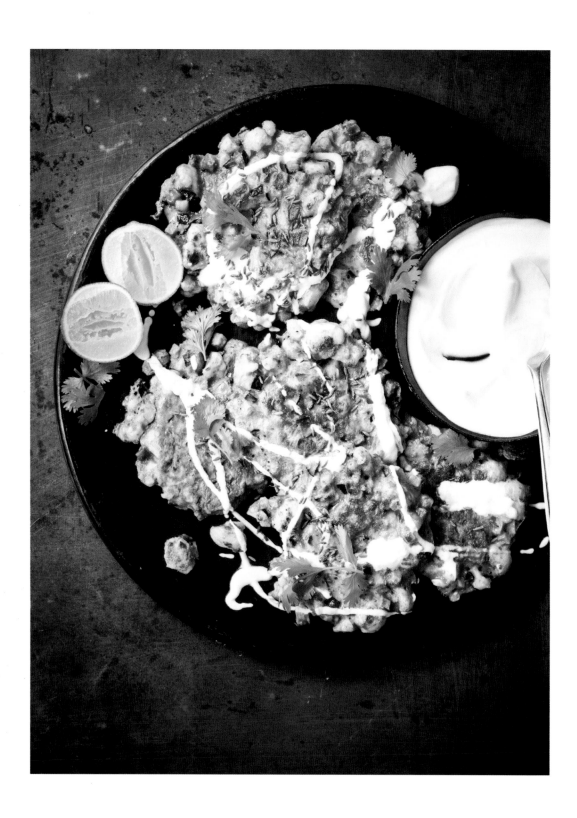

CAULIFLOWER AND AUBERGINE FRITTERS

These tasty fritters are great as a side dish or work wonderfully with dips. You wouldn't think you were eating vegetables — they feel like an indulgent treat, but don't have the downside.

SERVES 2

½ large cauliflower, cut into small florets

120g wholemeal flour

2 eggs, lightly beaten

1 garlic clove, crushed

1 tsp cumin seeds

1 tbsp coriander leaves, chopped

1 small aubergine, finely chopped

1 tbsp olive oil

120g Greek yoghurt (to serve)

1 lime, cut into wedges (to serve

1. Bring a large pot of water to the boil, add the cauliflower and cook for 5 minutes. Drain and set aside.

2. In a bowl, whisk together the flour, eggs, garlic, cumin seed and coriander leaves. Mix in the cauliflower and aubergine until well combined.

3. Heat the olive oil over a low-medium heat in a frying pan. Make 2–3 8cm rounds in the frying pan with the mixture, ensuring that they are well-spaced, and cook the fritters for 2–3 minutes on each side until golden brown.

4. Transfer the fritters on to a plate and serve with Greek yoghurt and lime wedges.

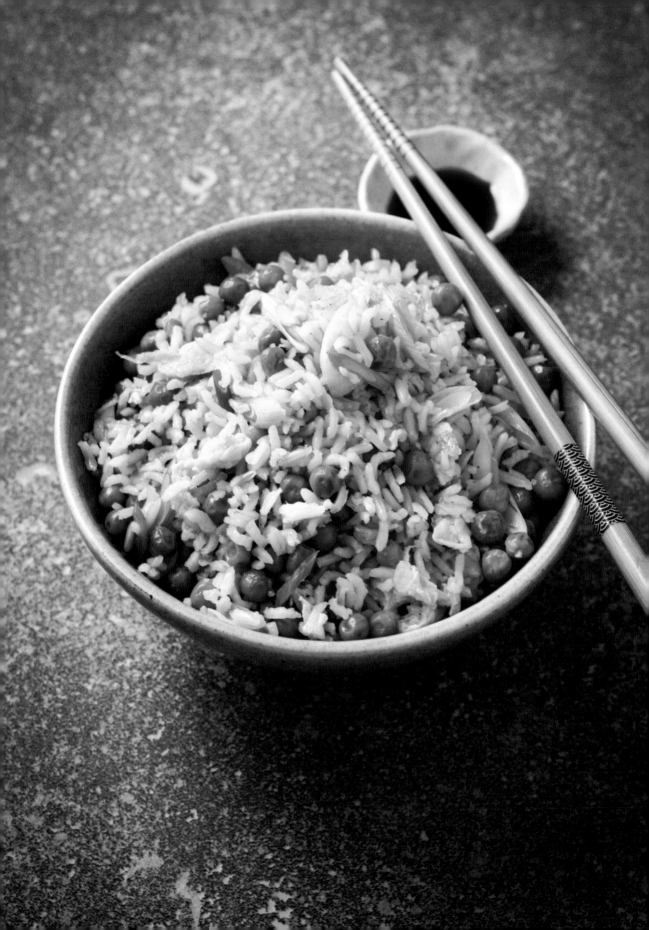

EGG FRIED RICE

This is a surprisingly balanced meal. When you think of egg fried rice you might think of greasy takeaway food, but this is much more nourishing and delicious.

SERVES 2

1 egg
1 tbsp sesame oil
1 tbsp olive oil
200g brown rice, cooked
1 tsp soy sauce
100g frozen peas
2 spring onions, finely chopped

1. Beat together the egg and sesame oil and set aside.

2. Heat the olive oil in a frying pan over a medium heat, and stir fry the rice for 3–4 minutes.

3. Add the soy sauce, peas and spring onions and continue to stir for another 3–4 minutes. Move the rice and vegetables to one side of the pan and add the egg to the other. Allow the egg to set for a few seconds, then toss with the rice.

4. Stir fry for another minute or so and serve straight away.

DINNER

FULL ENGLISH BREAKFAST

A traditional breakfast can actually be a perfectly balanced meal, so why not try eating one for dinner and using a different protein source? Here we use turkey bacon but you could try vegetarian sausages, burgers or chicken slices.

SERVES 2

2 tbsp olive oil
6 slices of turkey bacon
2 large tomatoes, halved
4 eggs
400g baked beans
2 slices of wholemeal toast

1. Heat 1 tablespoon of olive oil in a frying pan over a medium heat. Add the turkey bacon and tomatoes and fry for 5–10 minutes, turning the bacon occasionally.

2. At the same time, heat another frying pan with 1 tablespoon of olive oil over a medium heat. Crack the eggs into it and fry for 5 minutes, or until they are cooked to your liking.

3. Heat the baked beans in a saucepan or microwave.

4. Dish everything up in two servings, with a slice of toast per serving.

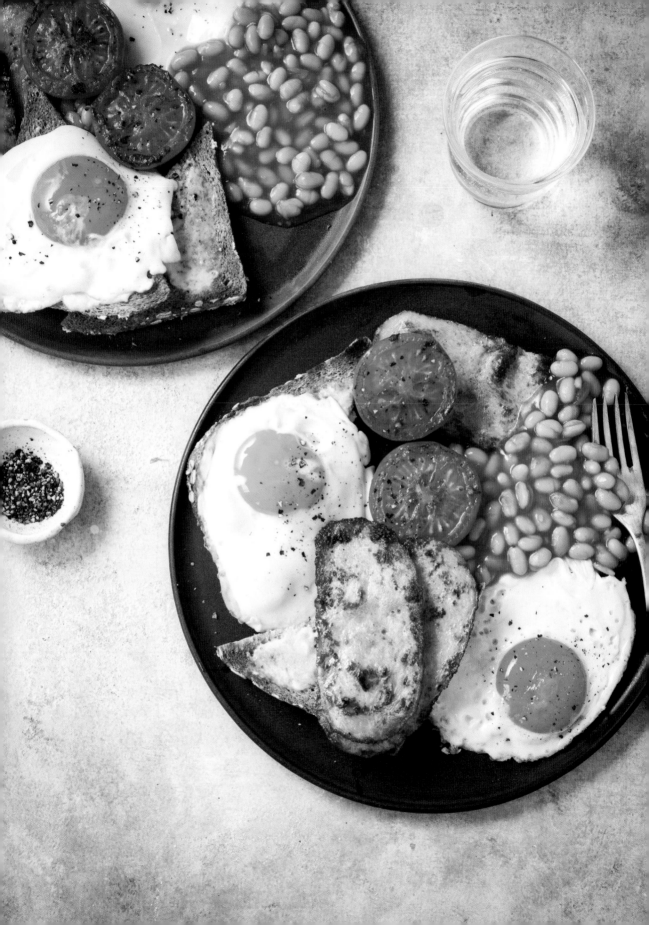

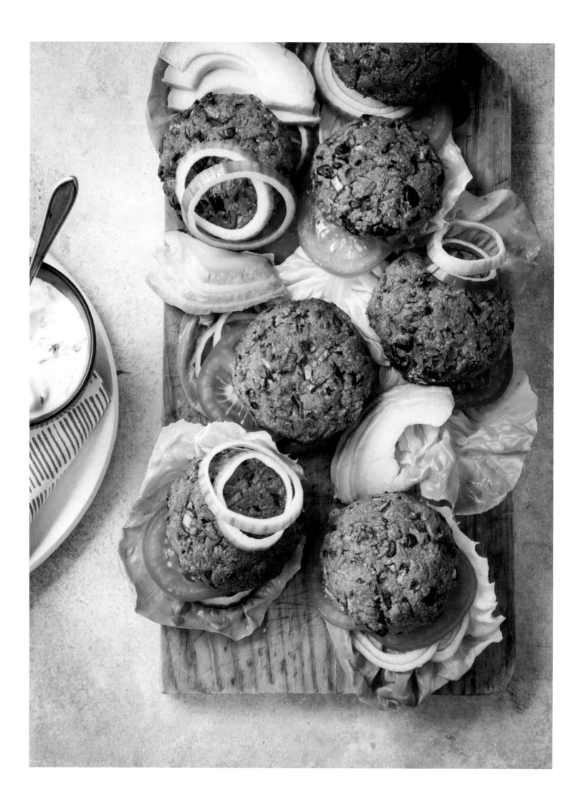

BEAN BURGERS

Bean burgers are super delicious and filling, so don't be put off by this veggie twist on a classic. You'll be amazed by the flavour in these burgers, plus you're getting some of your five a day! Enjoy with salad, potato wedges or a classic bun, you can't go wrong. You can freeze any leftover burgers in an airtight container.

MAKES 10 BURGERS

400g sweet potato, mashed

250g microwaveable brown rice

240g black beans, drained

150g red onion, finely diced

200g ground almonds

2 tsp ground cumin

1 tsp paprika

1 tsp sea salt

1 tsp ground pepper

Olive oil

1. Preheat the oven to 200°C/Fan 180°C/Gas Mark 6.

2. Cut the sweet potatoes in half and bake in the oven for 30 minutes, or until soft.

3. While the potatoes are cooking, cook the rice in the microwave for 1–2 minutes.

4. Add half the black beans to a mixing bowl and mash well. Then add the cooked sweet potato, rice, onion, ground almonds, spices, salt and pepper and mash again.

5. The mixture should be wet yet mouldable. Shape into 10 burgers.

6. Line a baking tray with baking paper, drizzle with a little olive oil and place the burgers onto the tray. Drizzle over a little more olive oil.

7. Bake the burgers for 35–40 minutes, carefully flipping them after 20 minutes. Remove from the oven and serve with a tomato and avocado salad.

CHINESE STIR FRY

Ronnie has picked up some terrific combinations of flavours while playing in China, and loves replicating them at home. A stir fry is a quick and simple meal and is packed with vegetables.

SERVES 4

For the marinade:

4 tbsp soy sauce

1 tbsp lemon juice

1 tbsp honey

1 tbsp sesame oil

½ tsp chilli flakes

4 chicken fillets, cut into strips

For the stir fry:

1 tbsp olive oil

2 garlic cloves, crushed

2 large carrots, peeled and thinly sliced

1 large green pepper, chopped

14 button mushrooms, sliced

160g broccoli, cut into florets

1 tbsp cornflour

320g brown rice, cooked

30g toasted sesame seeds (to serve)

1. In a bowl, whisk together all the ingredients for the marinade and add the chicken strips. Toss the chicken in to ensure it is coated, then leave in the fridge until needed.

2. Slice and chop the vegetables, and then heat the olive oil in a large saucepan over a medium-high heat.

3. Drain the chicken from the marinade (saving the leftover marinade) and cook for 5 minutes.

4. Add the garlic and cook for another minute or so. Add the carrots, pepper and mushrooms and continue to cook for 3–4 minutes. Then add the broccoli and cook for another 5 minutes.

5. Whisk the cornflour into the leftover marinade, and pour it into the pan. Bring to a simmer and cook for 5 minutes, until the mixture is thick.

6. Heat the cooked rice for 1 minute in the microwave and serve with the stir fry, finishing it with sesame seeds.

Simple veggie swap – switch chicken for tempeh.

PASTA WITH GARLIC PRAWNS

Having grown up in an Italian household, where garlic was added to everything, Ronnie is always keen to make it a main ingredient in his cooking. This is one of his signature dishes.

SERVES 1

100g wholemeal
penne pasta

1 tbsp olive oil

1 garlic clove, crushed

½ tsp dried chilli flakes

100g raw prawns,
peeled

1 tbsp lemon juice

2 tbsp parsley, chopped

Salt and pepper

1. Cook the pasta in a pan of boiling water, stirring occasionally until it is al dente. Drain and cover to keep warm.

2. While the pasta is boiling, heat the olive oil in a separate pan over a medium-high heat. Add the garlic and chilli flakes and stir for 1 minute. Add the prawns and cook for 4–5 minutes.

3. Add the cooked pasta to the pan and then the lemon juice and parsley.

4. Season and stir for another few minutes, and remove from the heat.

FISH PIE

A classic and satisfying dish for any occasion, a fish pie never fails to please a crowd. This recipe contains healthy fats, protein and carbs – it's a perfectly balanced meal.

SERVES 8

1½kg Maris Piper
potatoes
2 eggs
1 tbsp olive oil
50g unsalted butter
50g wholemeal flour
300ml fish stock
300ml milk of your
choice
3 bay leaves
50g mature Cheddar,
grated
2 tbsp lemon juice
300g boneless cod
200g salmon
(skin removed)
200g haddock
200g spinach

1. Preheat the oven to 200°C/Fan 180°C/Gas Mark 6.

2. Peel the potatoes and cut them into chunks. Boil in hot water for 15–20 minutes until soft, adding the eggs to the pan for the final 8 minutes. Remove the eggs, then peel and cut into quarters. Drain the potatoes and mash well with the olive oil. Set aside.

3. While the potatoes are boiling, make the sauce for the pie.

4. Melt the butter in a pan over a medium heat and stir in the flour. Add the fish stock gradually, stirring it in. Then add the milk and bay leaves, stirring until you have a silky sauce. Allow to cook for 10 minutes until it thickens. Stir in half the Cheddar and add the lemon juice. Stir until the cheese is melted and remove from the heat.

5. Slice the fish into chunks and spread them across a baking dish. Add the spinach.

6. Remove the bay leaves from the sauce and pour it over the fish. Add the eggs.

7. Spoon the potato over the pie filling and mash gently with a fork.

8. Bake in the oven for 35 minutes, then sprinkle over the remaining Cheddar and continue to bake until the fish is cooked and the potato is golden. Serve with green vegetables.

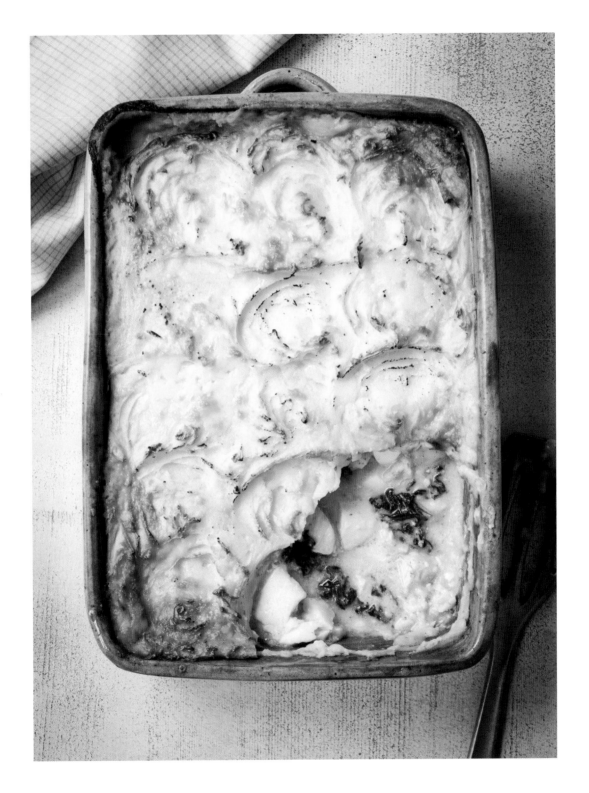

INDIAN CURRY

Ronnie loves curries and I've enjoyed working with him to create this mouth-watering dish that he can make at home. Serve with some rice or potatoes.

SERVES 4

1 tbsp olive oil

4 chicken fillet breasts, chopped into chunks

1 onion, finely chopped

2 garlic cloves, crushed

1 tsp ground coriander

½ tsp paprika

2 tbsp garam masala

400g tinned chopped tomatoes

200ml water

Salt and pepper

400g microwavable brown rice

To serve:

Coriander leaves

Lime wedges

Soured cream

1. Heat the oil in a large frying pan over a medium heat. Sear the chicken for 5 minutes and remove from the pan. Then fry the onion for about 5 minutes before adding the garlic and cooking for another minute.

2. Stir in the coriander, paprika and garam masala. Add the chunks of chicken back into the pan and cook for another 2 minutes, stirring occasionally to prevent them from sticking.

3. Add the chopped tomatoes and water. Season and allow to simmer for 10–15 minutes, until the chicken is cooked through. Remove from the heat.

4. Heat the rice and serve with the curry. Garnish with the coriander leaves, lime wedges and a dollop of soured cream.

Simple veggie swap – switch chicken for tofu.

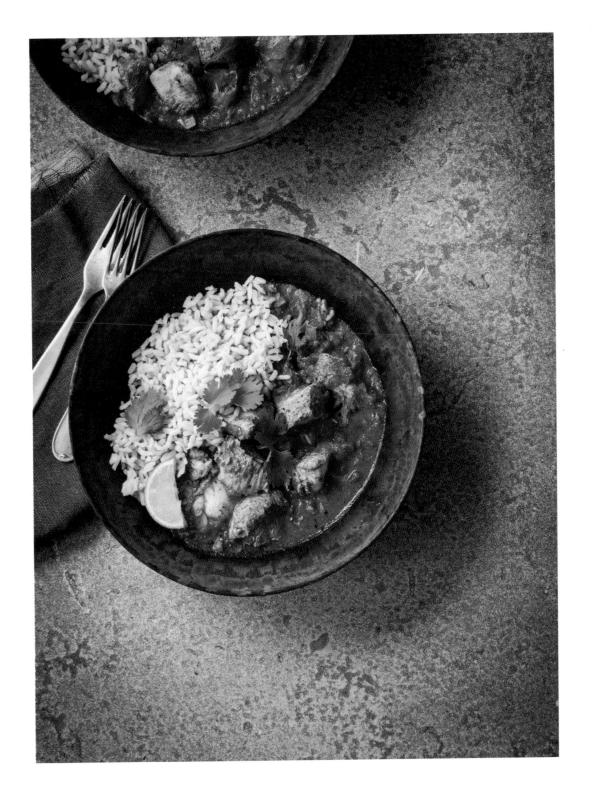

THAI FISHCAKES

Thai fishcakes have become a firm favourite in the UK, but they are often deep fried and coated in a heavy batter. This recipe has all the taste, yet none of the heaviness.

SERVES 2

350g cod fillet,
skinned and diced

1 spring onion, chopped

1 garlic clove, crushed

Zest of a lime

2 tsp red curry paste

1 tsp fresh ginger,
finely grated

1 egg

4 tbsp wholemeal flour

2 tbsp breadcrumbs

Salt and pepper

1 tbsp olive oil

1. Add the fish, spring onion, garlic, lime zest, curry paste, ginger and egg to a food processor and blend. Move the mixture to a bowl, stir in the flour and breadcrumbs, and season with salt and pepper.

2. Heat the oil in a frying pan over a medium heat. Mould the mixture into 4 burger shapes with your hands.

3. Cook the fishcakes two at a time, for 5–7 minutes on each side.

4. Remove from the heat and serve with green vegetables.

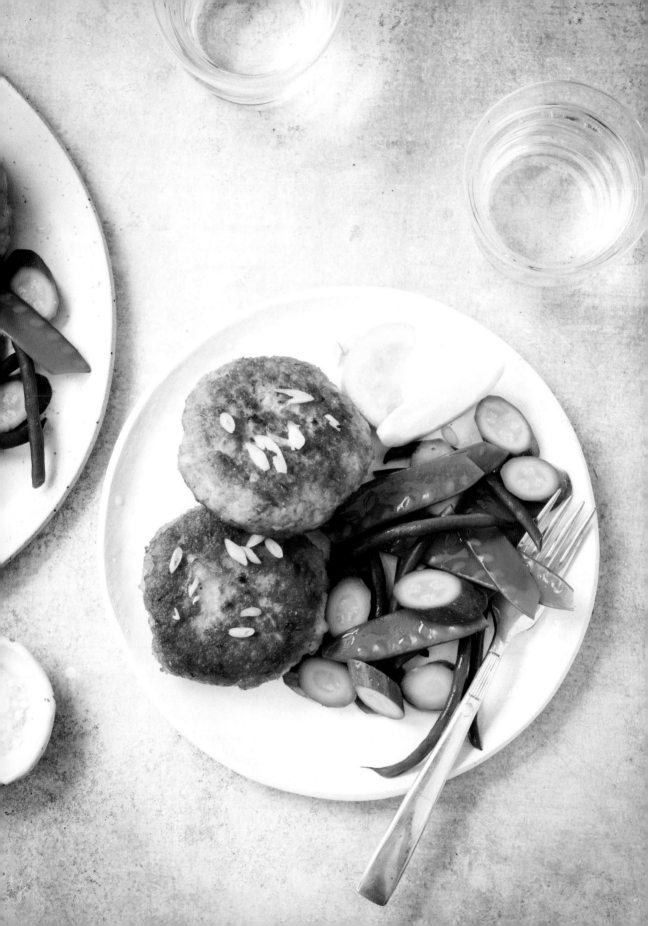

ROAST CHICKEN DINNER

Ronnie and I both adore a roast dinner on a Sunday. Despite common misconceptions, it can actually be both a balanced meal and a fantastic way of getting some vegetables into your diet. This is a slightly lighter take on the classic.

SERVES 4

600g potatoes,
peeled and halved

4 sprigs rosemary,
leaves picked

4 sprigs thyme,
leaves picked

2 tbsp olive oil

Salt and pepper

1 whole chicken
(approx 1.6kg)

500g baby carrots,
scrubbed

400g asparagus

1. Preheat the oven to 200°C/Fan 180°C/Gas Mark 6.

2. Place the potatoes in a large roasting tray and add the rosemary and thyme leaves. Drizzle with 1 tablespoon of olive oil, season with salt and pepper and toss well.

3. Rub the chicken with 1 tablespoon of olive oil and season, before placing it on top of the potatoes.

4. Roast in the oven for 40 minutes. Remove the tray from the oven and turn the potatoes. Add the carrots and return to the oven.

5. Cook for a further 25 minutes, then add the asparagus to the roasting tin. Cook for another 15 minutes, until the chicken is cooked through.

6. Remove the chicken from the tray and rest for 20 minutes. Keep the vegetables warm.

7. Carve the chicken and serve with the roast potatoes and vegetables.

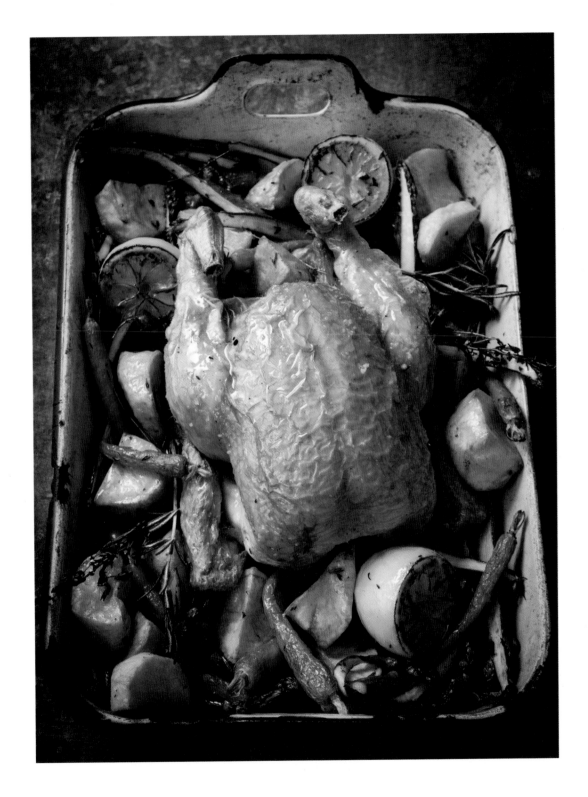

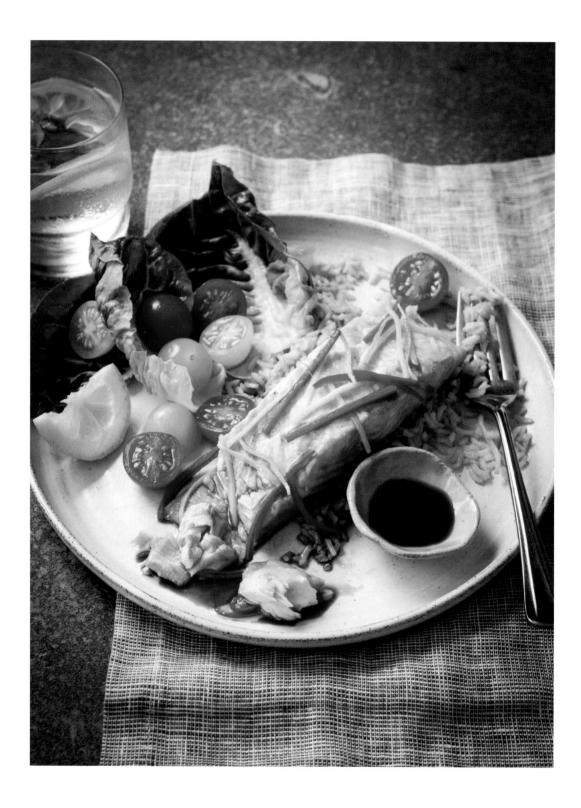

BAKED SALMON WITH FRESH CHILLI AND GINGER

The texture of salmon when it's baked in a tasty marinade is out of this world — and it also contains a good amount of healthy omega-3 fatty acids, which are fantastic for brain health.

SERVES 1

1 salmon fillet (180–220g)
1 tsp fresh ginger, julienned
½ fresh red chilli, thinly sliced
2 tbsp light soy sauce
80g baby gem lettuce
7 cherry tomatoes
½ lemon
100g microwaveable brown rice

1. Preheat the oven to 200°C/Fan 180°C/Gas Mark 6.

2. Place the salmon fillet on a large piece of foil on a baking tray and top with the ginger, chilli and soy sauce. Wrap the salmon in the foil and bake in the oven for 5–8 minutes.

3. Plate the lettuce and cut the tomatoes, squeezing the lemon juice on the salad. Heat the rice and plate with the salad.

4. Once the salmon is cooked, remove from the oven and serve with the salad and rice.

Simple veggie swap – switch salmon for tofu.

CHICKEN MILANESE

Succulent chicken and crunchy breadcrumbs are the components of a delicious chicken Milanese which, when paired with a refreshing green salad, makes for a great dinner.

SERVES 2

2 chicken breasts
90g wholemeal flour
½ tsp salt
½ tsp ground pepper
1 egg
70g breadcrumbs
2 tbsp olive oil
1 lemon, cut into wedges
Green salad (to serve)

1. Butterfly the chicken breasts, using a sharp knife. To do this, place the chicken breast on a chopping board, then slice into the side. Be careful not to cut all the way through. Next, open out the breast so that it resembles a butterfly.

2. Cover the chicken with Clingfilm and pummel with a rolling pin to even out the thickness.

3. Add the flour, salt and pepper to a small bowl and stir thoroughly. In another bowl, beat the egg. Place the breadcrumbs in a third bowl.

4. Place the first chicken breast in the bowl of flour. Make sure that both sides are covered, shake off any excess flour and then coat it in the egg. Finally, coat the chicken breast in the breadcrumbs.

5. Heat the olive oil in a frying pan over a medium-high heat. Place the coated chicken breasts in the pan and cook for 4–5 minutes on both sides, until they are cooked through and the breadcrumbs are golden brown.

6. Squeeze lemon over the chicken and serve with a green salad.

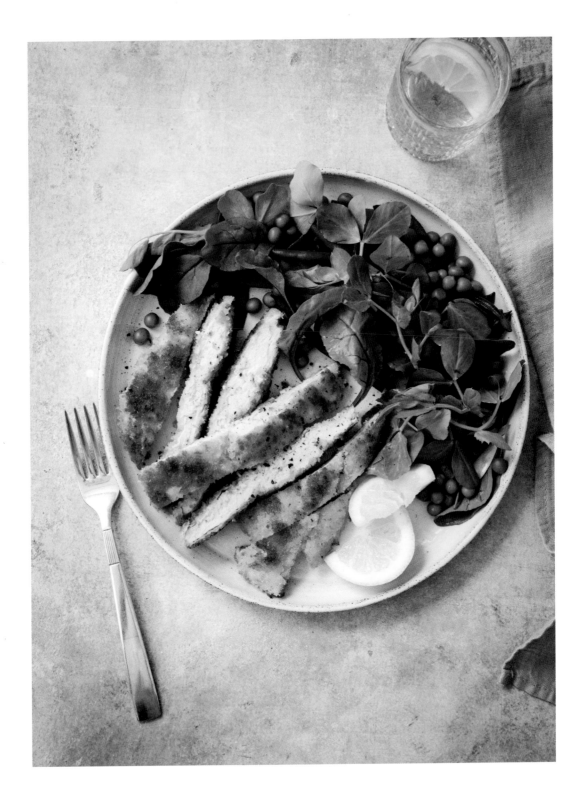

HEALTHY FISH AND CHIPS

*Fish and chips is a British favourite, but it doesn't have to be dripping in grease —
try this homemade take on the traditional version and you'll never look back.*

SERVES 2

400g Maris Piper
potatoes
1 tbsp olive oil
½ tsp salt
2 slices of wholemeal
bread
1 egg
2 haddock fillets
1 tbsp wholemeal flour
160g frozen peas
2 lemon wedges

1. Preheat the oven to 200°C/Fan 180°C/Gas Mark 6.

2. Peel the potatoes and chop into 'chunky chips'. Place them
   on a baking tray and drizzle with olive oil and toss in salt.
   Cook in the oven for 20 minutes, turning halfway through.

3. Lightly toast the bread, then pulse in a food processor to
   make breadcrumbs. Beat the egg in a bowl.

4. Place each fish fillet in the flour and, having coated both
   sides, shake off any excess and then coat it in the egg.
   Finally, coat the fish in the breadcrumbs and place the
   breaded fish on a lined baking tray and cook in the oven
   with the chips for a further 10 minutes.

5. 5 minutes before the fish and chips are ready, boil the peas
   for 3–4 minutes and then drain.

6. Remove the fish and chips from the oven, and serve with
   the peas and lemon wedge.

   Simple veggie swap – switch haddock for halloumi.

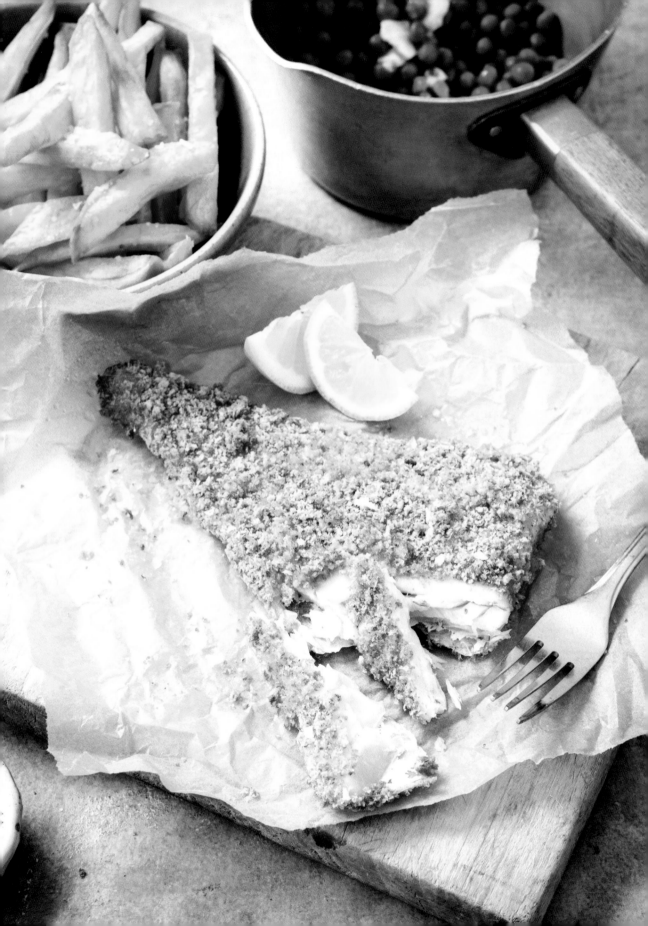

SINGAPORE NOODLES

Ronnie always orders a bowl of Singapore noodles when he goes out for a Chinese meal, so we've created our own version of this classic dish that contains less fat but just as much flavour.

SERVES 2

140g medium egg noodles

3 tbsp teriyaki sauce

2 tsp curry powder

1 tbsp olive oil

½ red pepper, chopped

½ green pepper, chopped

100g raw prawns, peeled

1 carrot, grated

1. Cook the noodles in a pot of boiling water, stirring to separate them. Drain and set aside.

2. In a small bowl, mix the teriyaki sauce and curry powder.

3. Heat the olive oil in a frying pan over a medium heat. Add the chopped peppers and cook for 2–3 minutes. Then add the prawns and cook for a further 5 minutes, before adding the noodles.

4. Stir for 2–3 minutes, then add the teriyaki sauce, curry powder mixture and the grated carrot. Continue to cook until the prawns are cooked through and divide into two servings.

Simple veggie swap – switch prawns for tempeh.

FIVE-MINUTE OPEN OMELETTE

The classic omelette is a healthy and affordable meal you can prepare in no time. Ronnie often gets home late and this is one of his go-to meals after a busy day – it's nutritious but not so heavy that he can't eat it late at night.

SERVES 1

1 tbsp olive oil
3 eggs, beaten
A handful of spinach
½ red pepper, chopped

1. Heat the olive oil in a frying pan over a medium-high heat and pour in the eggs.

2. Allow to cook until the sides of the omelette start to set – you can tilt the pan to move the mixture around to encourage it to cook more quickly. Add the spinach and peppers, and continue to cook for another few minutes.

3. When the middle of the omelette is set, use a spatula to slide it on to a plate.

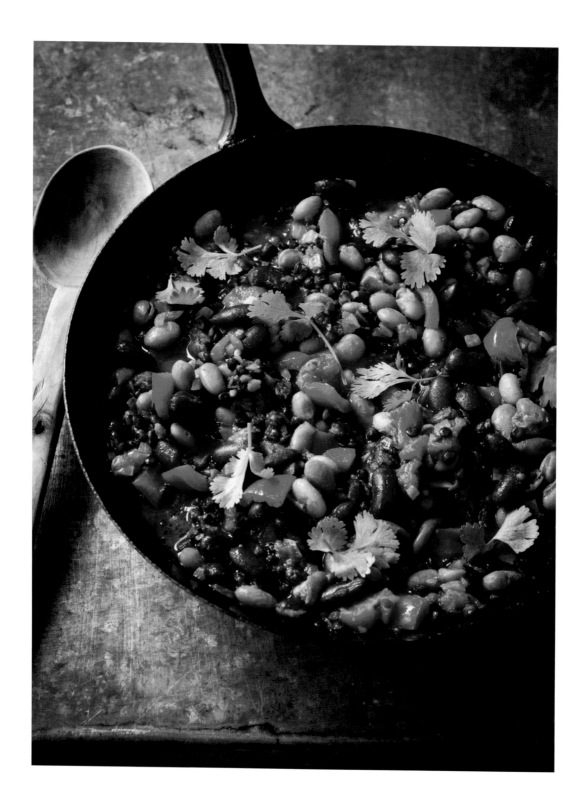

VEGAN CHILLI

This delicious and comforting chilli is suitable for the whole family. It's full of fibre, terrific for a healthy gut and will leave you feeling full and satisfied. Try adding a dollop of Greek yoghurt for some additional protein.

SERVES 2

1 tbsp olive oil

1 clove garlic, crushed

½ onion, finely chopped

1 red pepper, diced

200g tinned chopped tomatoes

50ml vegetable stock

1 tsp chilli powder

200g pinto beans, drained

200g kidney beans, drained

200g puy lentils, cooked

100ml water

Coriander leaves (to garnish)

1. Heat the olive oil in a sacuepan over a medium heat and add the garlic, onion and pepper.

2. Then add the chopped tomatoes, vegetable stock and chilli powder and cook for 5 minutes, stirring occasionally. Add the pinto beans, kidney beans, lentils and water and simmer for 10 minutes.

3. Remove from the heat, split into 2 servings and garnish with coriander leaves.

VEGAN THAI CURRY

Thai curries are great when you want to cook an easy-yet-decadent dish – the rich coconut milk and the flavours of the spices and vegetables make it completely delicious. It's dairy-free and contains plant-based protein from peas and edamame beans, which makes for a vegan-friendly, balanced dish.

SERVES 2

3 small potatoes, quartered
2 tbsp olive oil
½ onion, finely chopped
½ tsp ground ginger
1 tbsp green curry paste
250ml coconut milk
250g tofu, cut into cubes
100g frozen peas
1 tsp rice wine vinegar
A handful of spinach
30g sesame seeds
½ red chilli, thinly sliced

1. Boil the potatoes in a saucepan of water for 10 minutes, drain and set aside.

2. While the potatoes are boiling, make the sauce.

3. Heat 1 tablespoon of olive oil in a small saucepan over a medium heat and add the onion. Cook for 3–4 minutes, then add the ginger, curry paste and coconut milk. Bring the sauce to a simmer.

4. In a small frying pan, heat 1 tablespoon of olive oil and add the tofu. Cook until it is golden.

5. Add the peas and potatoes to the curry sauce, and then add the cooked tofu. Stir for 1–2 minutes, before adding the rice wine vinegar and spinach.

6. Top with sesame seeds and sliced chill to serve.

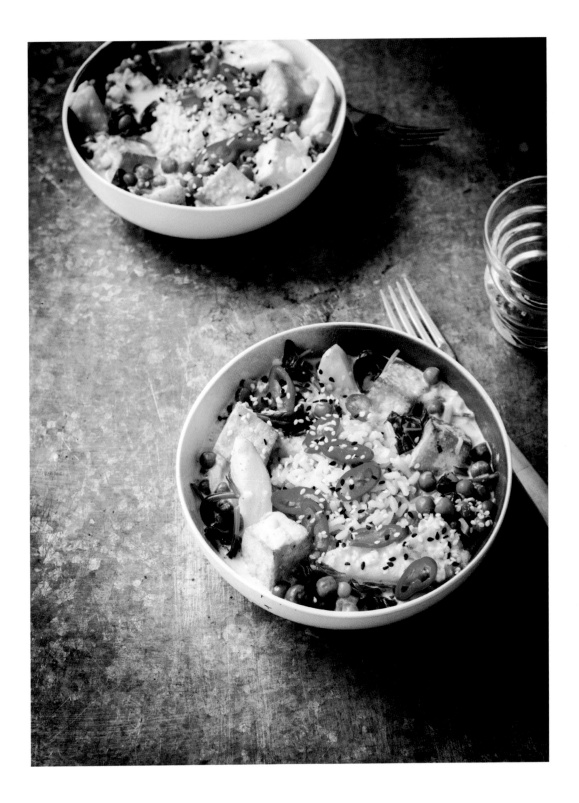

TOMATO AND MOZZARELLA PASTA BAKE

Cooking doesn't have to be complicated – you can buy a can of tomato and basil sauce from any supermarket as a cheap and healthy way of stocking your kitchen cupboards with versatile items. This pasta bake is simple to make, and very tasty.

SERVES 1

100g wholemeal penne pasta

125g tomato and basil sauce

40g cherry tomatoes, quartered

30g mozzarella, torn

1. Preheat the oven to 200°C/Fan 180°C/Gas Mark 6.

2. Boil the pasta in a large saucepan of boiling salted water until al dente, stirring occasionally. Drain and rinse well.

3. Pour the pasta into an oven-safe dish and stir in the tomato and basil sauce, and the tomatoes.

4. Add the mozzarella, dotting it over the pasta.

5. Bake in the oven for 15–20 minutes, until it is crispy on top.

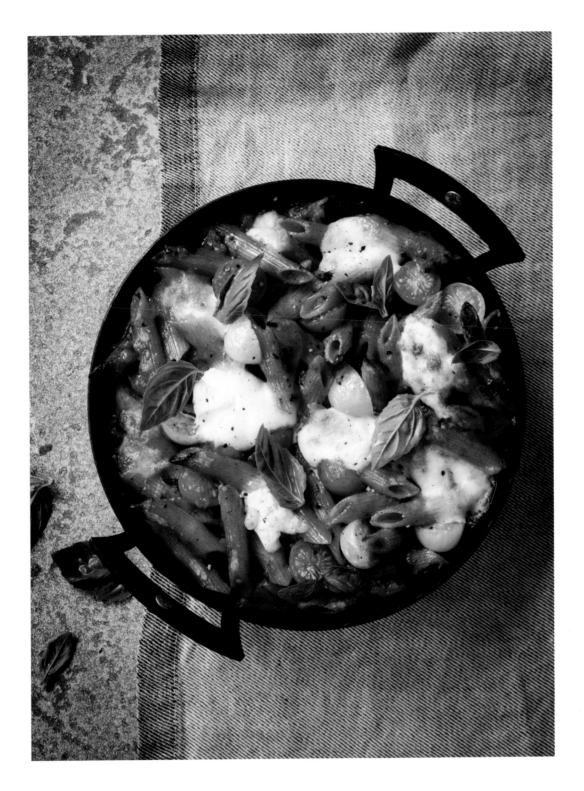

ON-THE-GO SNACKS

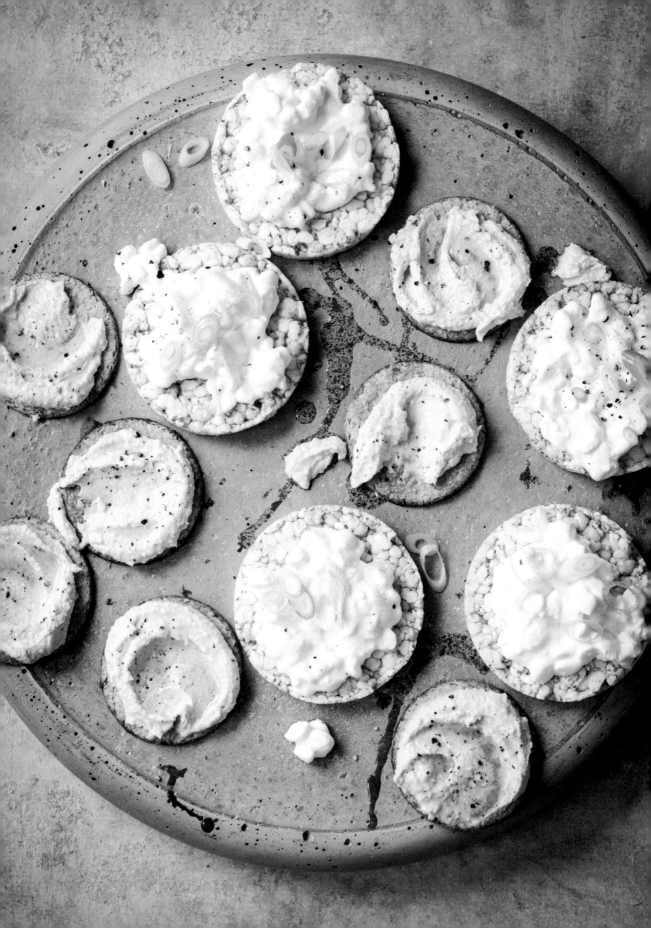

OATCAKES AND HUMMUS

You can grab a pot of hummus and pack of oatcakes from any supermarket –
this is a snack that contains lots of fibre, protein and healthy fats.

SERVES 1

60g hummus
3 oatcakes

1. Hummus is the perfect snack, being a good source of protein, and provides essential minerals such as manganese, copper and iron.

2. Spread the hummus evenly across the oatcakes.

RICE CAKES WITH COTTAGE CHEESE

Ronnie likes to keep some cottage cheese in his fridge at all times, so I
encouraged him to start spreading it on rice cakes to make sure he gets
carbohydrates with his protein.

SERVES 1

200g cottage cheese
3 rice cakes
1 spring onion, sliced

1. Cottage cheese is an excellent source of protein and is also high in calcium.

2. Spread the cottage cheese on the rice cakes and garnish with the spring onions.

BRITISH EGG MUFFINS

Egg muffins are delicious and wholesome – the muffins contain lots of fibre and the scrambled eggs are full of protein.

SERVES 1

2 eggs
1 tbsp olive oil
Salt and pepper
1 wholemeal muffin, toasted

1. Eggs are an excellent source of high-quality protein and contain essential nutrients including vitamins A, D, B12 and selenium.

2. Beat the eggs in a bowl. Heat the olive oil in a saucepan over a medium-high heat and pour in the eggs. Season with salt and pepper.

3. Gently scramble the eggs with a spatula. Cook for 2–3 minutes until the eggs begin to set.

4. Serve the eggs on top of the muffin.

   Simple vegan swap – switch eggs for tofu.

For the tofu:
115g tofu
1 tsp turmeric
1tsp smoked paprika

1. If using tofu, chop it up and use a fork to crumble the pieces into bite-sized chunks.

2. Pour some olive oil into a frying pan and, when it's hot, add the tofu. I like to throw in some turmeric and smoked paprika for extra flavour, too.

3. Stir until combined and cook over a medium-high heat for 5–10 minutes, stirring occasionally.

4. Serve the tofu on top of the muffin.

AVOCADO AND EGGS

Ronnie and I both love breakfast, so I devised a list of snacks that he can whip up at a moment's notice. This brunch-inspired snack provides the perfect combination of fats, carbohydrates and protein!

SERVES 1

2 eggs
Salt and pepper
1 tbsp olive oil
½ avocado, sliced

1. Beat the eggs in a bowl and add salt and pepper. Heat the olive oil in a frying pan over a medium-high heat and pour in the eggs.

2. Gently scramble the eggs with a spatula. Cook for 2–3 minutes, until the eggs begin to set.

3. Serve the eggs on a plate with the avocado.

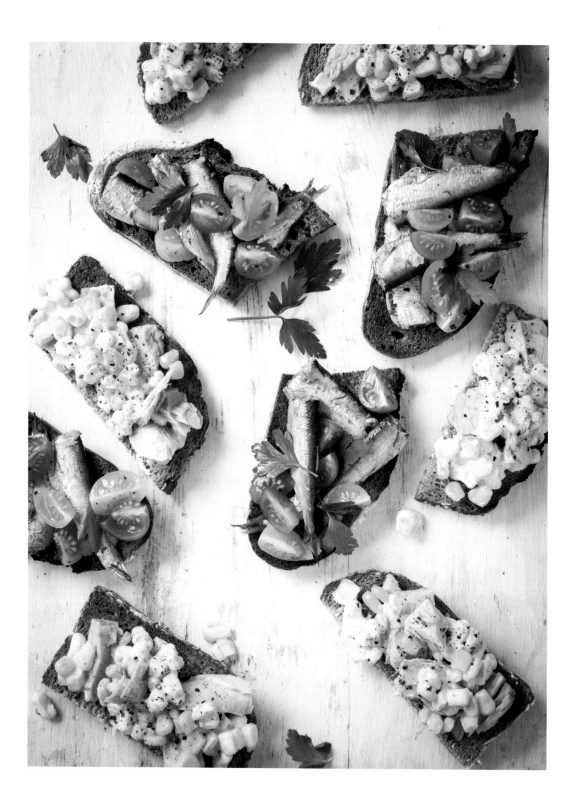

RYE BREAD WITH TUNA AND SWEETCORN

This perfect snack is a delicious and simple combination of tuna and sweetcorn that doesn't contain any mayonnaise. The textured rye bread is a delicious addition, too. High in protein, tuna is also a good source of omega-3 fatty acids.

SERVES 1

80g tinned sweetcorn
100g tinned tuna
1 slice of rye bread, toasted

1. Drain the sweetcorn and the tuna, then gently mash them together. Serve on toasted rye bread.

SARDINES ON TOAST

This recipe takes me and Ronnie back to our childhoods when our grandparents would serve toast with sardines, a meal that was always satisfying, healthy and delicious. Sardines are a fabulous source of omega-3 fatty acids, calcium, iron and potassium.

SERVES 1

100g sardines
1 slice of wholemeal bread, toasted
Cherry tomatoes, quartered (to serve)

1. Place the sardines on the toast and top with the quartered cherry tomatoes.

OAT SMOOTHIE

A smoothie is a great way to top up your nutrients throughout the day. A top tip is to always have a jar of oats in the cupboard and fruit such as peeled bananas and berries in the freezer, so you are always ready to blend.

SERVES 1

50g oats

1 banana

200ml milk of your choice

½ tsp cinnamon

5 ice cubes

1. Blend all the ingredients in a blender and pour into a glass.

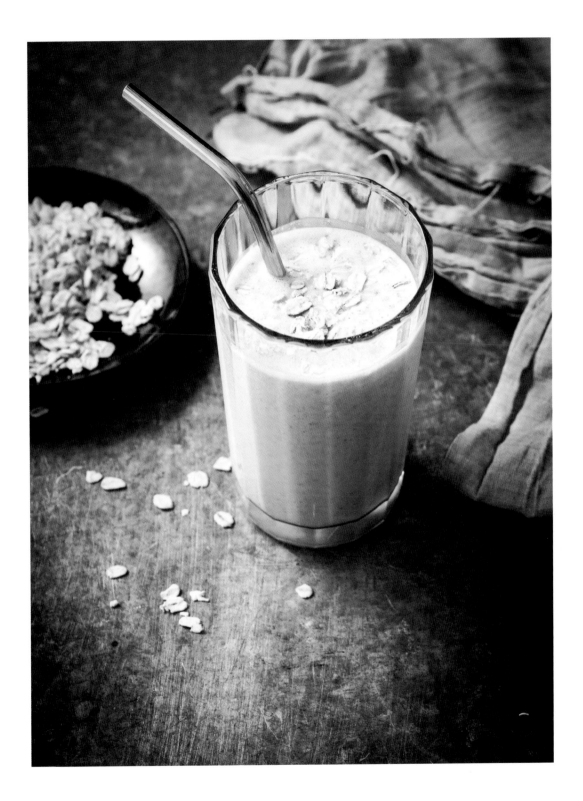

YOGHURT AND BERRIES WITH NUT BUTTER

Greek yoghurt is a great source of protein and also contains beneficial live bacteria. When paired with the healthy fats in nut butter and the vitamins from berries, this is a great snack to have in-between meals when you need a pick-me-up.

SERVES 1

80g Greek yoghurt
30g raspberries
30g blueberries
20g dried cranberries
2 tbsp nut butter
of your choice

1. Place the yoghurt in a bowl and scatter the berries on top. Serve with 2 tablespoons of your favourite nut butter.

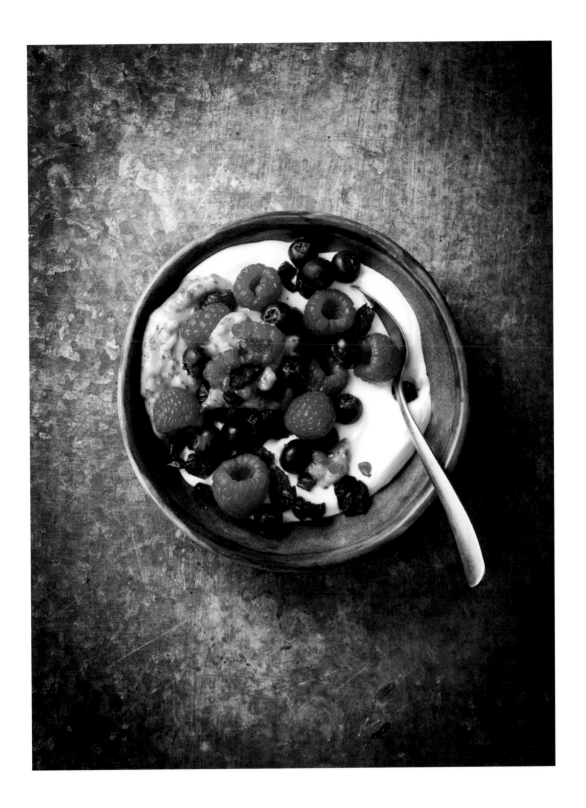

NUTS

A handful of nuts is a simple and nourishing snack — you should always have a pack in your bag for moments when you're hungry while on the go. Try a different variety of nuts each time.

SERVES 1

40g nuts of your choice

Nuts are a great source of dietary fibre and provide a variety of vitamins, including several B vitamins (such as folate). They are also a good way to get vitamin E and minerals including calcium, iron, zinc, potassium and magnesium into your diet.

Eat as a snack between meals.

BANANA AND NUTS

This is a great snack and perfect to eat on the go. Measuring out the nuts, wrapping them in tin foil and keeping them in your bag is a great idea.

SERVES 1

30g walnuts
1 banana

Banana and nuts are a great source of carbohydrates and protein that will keep you full of energy until your next meal.

INDEX

(page numbers in *italics* refer to photographs)

addiction 10, 20, 23
almond milk, benefits of 42
antioxidants 88
anxiety 62
appetite hormones 74
Apricot Overnight Oats *144*, 145
asparagus 186
aubergines 87, 166, 169
avocados 41, 49, 94, 95, 99, 108, 131, 157, 207
Avocado and Eggs 207

Baked Fish with Herbs 155
Baked Salmon with Fresh Chilli and Ginger *188*, 189
Banana and Cinnamon Breakfast Cookies *126*, 127
Banana and Nuts 215
Banana Bread *128*, 129
Banana Porridge 110
bananas 92, 108, 110, 113, 116, 124, 127, 129, 136, 139, 140, 210, 215
Bean Burgers *176*, 177
beans 37, 40, 83, 152, 154, 174, 177, 197
berry fruits 92, 108, 111, 116, 120, 124, 133, 136, 139, 140, 212
Berry Porridge 111
Berry Smoothie *138*, 139
bingeing 13
Black Bean Burritos 152, *153*

blood glucose, 'spike' in 61, 62
blood sugar 61–3
brain:
    carbohydrates benefit 30
    gains 48–9
    glucose fuels 62
    and gut health 96
    health 79–80
    'second' 80
breakfast, benefits of 43, 46
Breakfast Omelette 122, *123*
Breakfast Pancakes 116, *117*
Breakfast Pitta Sandwich 135
British Egg Muffins 206
burgers 177

calories, explained 60
carbohydrates 30, 41, 48, 57, 61–3, 64–6, 79
Carrot Cake Overnight Oats *144*, 145
carrots 145, 186
Cauliflower and Aubergine Fritters *168*, 169
charcoal 91
cheese 114, 122, 135, 149, 152, 163, 200, 205
Cheese Porridge 114
Chia Seed Raspberry Jam on Toast 120, *121*
chia seeds 120, 139, 141, 142
chicken *81*, 150, 159, 160, 165, 182, 186, 190
    benefits of 40, 79, *80*

Chicken Kebabs *158*, 159
Chicken Milanese 190, *191*
Chicken Salad Sandwich with Greek
  Yoghurt 160, *161*
Chinese Stir Fry 178
Chocolate and Coconut Overnight Oats
  143
Chocolate Porridge *112*, 113
Cinnamon Muesli *132*, 133
Cinnamon Spice Overnight Oats 142
Classic Overnight Oats 141
cod 95, 155, 180, 184
coeliac disease 89
complex carbohydrates 61–2, 65
cranberries 133, 160, 212
cravings 61
cross-contamination 89

Davis, Steve 25
depression 28, 62, 80, 99
dessert, what to eat for 45
diet plan 39
dieting, pitfalls of 34, 53
dinner, when to eat 45, 46

eating-out plate 72
Egg Fried Rice *170*, 171
Egg Muffins 115, 206
exercise 52, 74, 77, 78

Falafel 83
fatigue 16, 62, 64, 69, 97
fats 41, 49, 68, 79
fibre 61, 66
Fish and Chips 192, *193*
Fish Fillet 87
Fish Pie 180, *181*

fitness plate 72, 92
5-a-day 41, 42, 75
Five-minute Open Omelette 195
Flatbread and Hummus 134
flaxseed 31, 43, 92, 139
focus, how to 42
folates 37
French Toast 124, *125*
Fresh Breakfast Bowl 108, *109*
Fruit Salad 84
Full English Breakfast 174, *175*

Gingerbread Porridge 113, *112*
glucose 32, 62
gluten 89
glycogen 59, 64, 67
go-to carbohydrates 48
goal-setting 31, 54, 74
grains 39, 41, 61–3, 65, 89, 91
Granola *118*, 119
grazing 67
Green Smoothie 136, *137*
gut health 80, 89–91, 96
gut-health plate 72, 86–7

haddock 95, 180, 192
Healthy Fish and Chips 192, *193*
'healthy' options, beware of 99
Hendry, Stephen 21, 23
Hummus 83, 205
hydration 43, 69

Indian Curry 182, *183*
iron deficiency 37
irritability 37, 62

Jacket Sweet Potato and Homemade
   Beans 154

kefir 88
kimchi 88
kitchen tips 100
knowledge, as 'magic ingredient' 30
kombucha 88

Lambert, Rhiannon 13–15, 25, 62, 68, 69,
   86, 96, 102
      Ronnie first meets 29–30, 39, 53
lentils 40, 63, 197
low-carb diet 52, 66
lunch, benefits of 44, 46

mackeral 86
macronutrients 68, 79
mangoes 139, 140, 157
Mango, Prawn and Avocado Salad 156,
   157
mental health 24, 29, 36, 72
mental-health plate 72
metabolism 60, 66
micronutrients 80, 84
milk:
      benefits of 32, 42, 43, 57, 92
      fermented 88
      plant-based 98
mindful eating 32–9, 96–7
Miso Aubergine 87, 166, 167
monounsaturates 68, 80
mood plate 72
mood swings 61, 62, 64
motivation 12, 54
muscle-building 67
mushrooms 115, 122, 165, 178

neurodegenerative diseases 80
niacin deficiency 37
non-coeliac gluten sensitivity 89
non-starchy foods 78
noodles 194
nutrient intake 56, 57, 60
nuts and seeds, benefits of 41, 214

Oat Smoothie 210, 211
Oatcakes and Hummus 204, 205
oats 92, 108, 110, 111, 113, 114, 119, 127,
   133, 136, 140, 141, 142, 143, 145, 210
olive oil, benefits of 41, 68, 79, 80, 81
omega-3 68, 80, 110, 189, 209
Omelette 195
O'Sullivan, Ronnie:
      head-butting suspension 21
      physical-health problems 29, 52
      Rhiannon first meets 29–30, 39, 53
      running taken up by 10, 20, 21, 23, 30,
         39, 54, 64, 74, 77
      as Snooker World Champion 21, 25

Pasta Bake 200, 201
Pasta with Garlic Prawns 179
Peanut Butter Smoothie 136, 137
peas 165, 171, 192, 198
performance, how to maximise 57
Peters, Steve 21
Pizza Wraps 162, 163
plates, what to put on 31, 72, 75, 79–80,
   81
Poached Eggs on Rye Bread with
   Avocado 130, 131
Porridge, Walnut, Berries, Almond Milk &
   Flaxseed 92
potatoes 180, 186, 192, 198

prawns 157, 179, 194
pre-tournament plate 72, 94–5
probiotics 87, 88, 91
processed foods, minimising 60
protein 40, 43, 57, 67, 79, 111

Rainbow Chilli Stir Fry 150, *151*
Reardon, Ray 25
rice 31, 32, 41, 46, 48, 59, 61, 63, 65, 70,
    84, 171, 177, 178, 182
Rice Cakes with Cottage Cheese *204*,
    205
Rice Salad 84
on-the-road plate 72, 82–3
Roast Chicken Dinner 186, *187*
Roasted Fish with Baked Sweet Potato
    94–5
roasted vegetables, benefits of 80, *81*,
    95
Ronnie and Rhiannon's Homemade
    Pizza *148*, 149
Ronnie's Paella *164*, 165
running 98
    extra nutrition for 54
    foods to eat *after* 59
    foods to eat *before* 57
Rye Bread with Tuna and Sweetcorn
    208, 209

salmon 86, 180, 189
sardines 209
Sardines on Toast *208*, 209
Sauerkraut Salad 87, 88
sea bass 95
seeds and nuts benefits of 41, 80, 214
selenium 37, 206
Singapore Noodles 194

snacking 43–4, 46
snooker depression 99
spinach 108, 115, 122, 135, 136, 163, 180,
    195, 198
Strawberry Mango Smoothie 140
sugar, cutting down on 60, 98
sweet potato 80, 94, 95, 154, 177

Thai Curry 198, *199*
Thai Fishcakes 184, *185*
thiamin deficiency 37
Tomato and Mozzarella Pasta Bake 200,
    201
Tomato and Mozzarella Pizza Wraps
    162, 163
training day plate 72
training programme 64, 77
Tropical Smoothie *138*, 139
tuna 209
type 2 diabetes 66

Vegan Chilli *196*, 197
Vegan Thai Curry 198, *199*
Vegetable Sticks 84
vitamins and minerals 32, 36, 37, 54, 80,
    88, 209

water-soluble vitamins 54

yo-yo weight change 13, 20
yoghurt, benefits of 31, 43, 45, 57, 84, 88
Yoghurt and Berries with Nut Butter 212,
    213

RHIANNON LAMBERT

Rhiannon is a Registered Nutritionist (RNutr) specialising in weight management and sports nutrition. Founder of leading Harley Street clinic Rhitrition and bestselling author of *Re-Nourish: A Simple Way To Eat Well*, Rhiannon's qualified approach to nutrition and total dedication to her clients' needs has seen her work with some of the world's most influential people. Having worked with Olympic athletes, Rhiannon demonstrates the dramatic impact nutrition can have on performance at the highest level.

Rhiannon has obtained a first-class Bachelor's (BSc) degree in Nutrition and Health and a Masters (MSc) degree in Obesity, Risks and Prevention. She is also a Master Practitioner in Eating Disorders and Obesity, having obtained a diploma from The National Centre For Eating Disorders, approved by The British Psychological Society (BPS). Rhiannon continuously furthers her study, becoming a Personal Trainer and delving into the world of pre and post natal nutrition.

Rhiannon hosts the leading nutrition and health podcast, *Food For Thought*, and is pioneering in the world of social media via her @rhitrition platforms. Regularly seen in the press contributing to the latest health news, 'in a world full of confusing nutritional advice, Rhiannon Lambert is a beacon of sense' say *The Independent*.

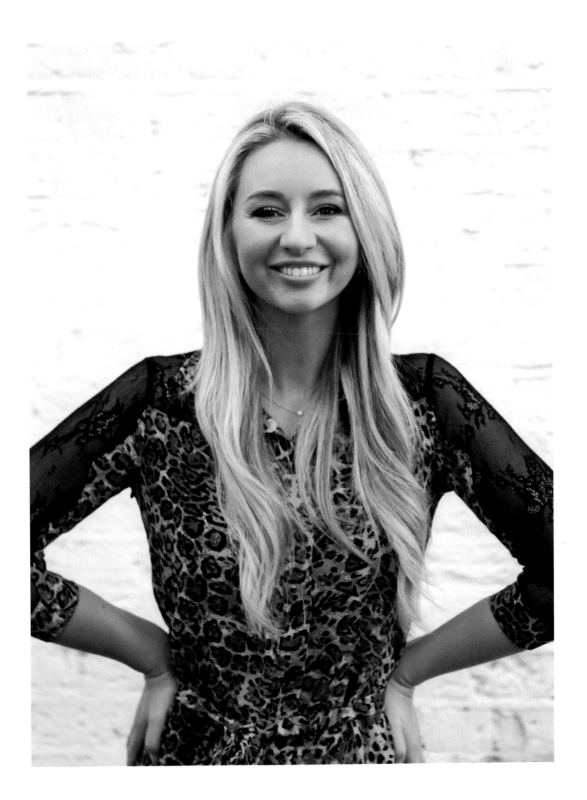

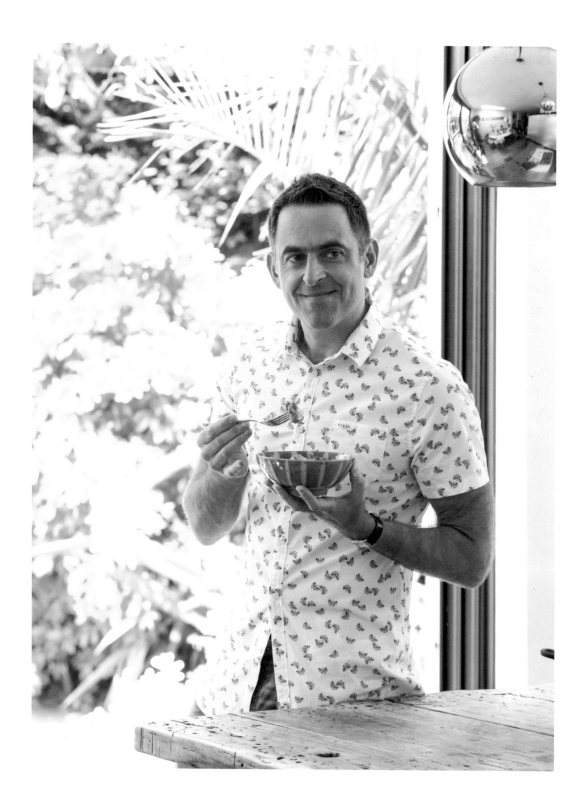

RONNIE O'SULLIVAN

Ronnie O'Sullivan OBE is the world's most popular snooker player, and one of the greatest sportsmen ever to enter the game. First picking up a cue at just 7 years old and winning his first ranking title just ten years later, Ronnie has won an incredible 34 ranking titles. His achievements include an exceptional 5 World Titles, a record 7 UK Championships, and a record 7 Masters Titles - setting another record of 19 titles in Triple Crown tournaments.

Ronnie is widely considered to be one of the most naturally gifted players the game has ever seen. A right-handed player, he can also play to an extremely high standard with his left hand. He is a born showman and a firm favourite among the crowds.

Away from snooker, Ronnie loves running and cooking, which made *Top of Your Game* the perfect project for him. Previously, Ronnie found himself over-exercising, eating badly, and lacking energy, but thanks to his new attitude towards his physical and mental health, he continues to excel in his sport over 25 years since turning professional.

ACKNOWLEDGEMENTS

Since learning about food, I feel better than ever. Making those changes came once I understood that what I put into my body helps me get the absolute best out of it.

I want to share that message and knowledge with all of you to make sure you feel the best you can as well. I hope this book can be your starting point because we can only do better once we know what to do. So, the first thank you I want to make is to Rhiannon, for educating me on how important nutrition is. Eating well and getting control over my diet has given me the energy I need to keep fit and maintain a healthy mind and body. Learning all she had to teach me has truly changed my life; I won't ever look back.

I'd also like to thank my partner, Laila. Making big changes to your lifestyle is hard at the start and I couldn't have done it without her support. I am so lucky to have a partner who has the same vision and goals as me. She knows how important it is to look after yourself and has been behind me 100% on this. We make a great team.